VINEGAR SOCKS

VINEGAR SOCKS

Traditional Home Remedies
for Modern Living

KARIN BERNDL
& NICI HOFER

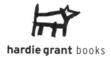

hardie grant books

To Regina, Herbert and Sieglinde.

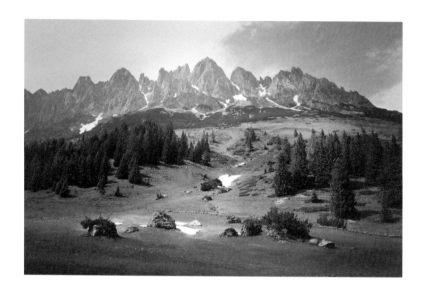

Hochkönig, Austria 2012

CONTENTS

INTRODUCTION

Whenever we suggest to our non-Austrian friends that the best way to treat a cold is with a home remedy, we're usually greeted with disbelief and amusement. After years of encountering this reaction, we decided that the time was right to share some of our mums' recipes from our childhood memories and those we have collected, and arrange them neatly in this book. We hope that they will keep you entertained whilst your body is on its way to feeling better.

We both grew up in Austria where no herb or vegetable was too strange to be applied or consumed to help the body heal. During our childhoods, we took it for granted that natural healing was used to cure common ailments. Now, as adults, we know how fortunate we were. 'Vinegar socks' is probably the best-known traditional fever-cure in Austria, and we doubt there is an Austrian who hasn't heard of it.

Medicine in the last few thousand years has seen some rather interesting trends. Quite some time ago, plants and roots were all there was, doing the trick for no one less famous than Queen of Sheba and Cleopatra — see, not just great eye make-up — these trendsetters! Then religion was believed to heal and cure, followed by potions. The trusty snake oil salesman delivered a great pitch, for sure, but only until people called his bluff and moved on to pills - which were quickly replaced by antibiotics. So today, did we come full circle and realised that the power of plants, herbs, seeds and vegetables in combination with hundreds of years of old techniques can help us heal naturally? We do think so! The world seems ready for what has survived for so many generations in a little Alpine country: Vinegar Socks!

BEFORE
YOU START ...

CHOOSE ORGANIC

Ingredients should always be organic, natural and preferably bought in a reputable health food store, an organic market or pharmacy. If you have a garden or a window sill, ingredients can be easily homegrown. If any of the ingredients are not available locally, they can be sourced online through reputable farmers or websites.

THE FRESHER, THE BETTER

Always prepare the recipes with fresh ingredients. You can store some of the remedies in the fridge for up to a couple of days, but they are most potent when used immediately after preparation. If the recipe calls for you to heat ingredients, never use a microwave.

DRYING YOUR HERBS

We have used dried and fresh herbs in our photographs, but you can use whatever you have available.

Wash your herbs or blossoms gently. Find a dry and warm place away from direct sunlight and prepare the surface with baking paper or a cotton tea towel. Arrange the herbs on the area so they dry evenly. This usually takes about 1 week. When the leaves crumble easily, they are ready to be stored, preferably in a glass or ceramic jar. Don't crush the leaves until you are ready to use them. The stored leaves can last for up to a year.

HOW TO STERILIZE A JAR

Wash the jar and lid in hot, soapy water. Next, boil the jar in a large pan for 10–15 minutes. Remove with tongs and pour any remaining water out of the jar. Place the jar in a safe spot without drying it. We pour boiling water over the inside of the lid to avoid damage to the seal, but make sure the lid you use is not corroded.

VINEGAR SOCKS

Traditionally used in
Austria to lower fever

This home remedy is one most of us in Austria would have come across as children. As we lay sick in bed, our mums would have applied these socks to our feet — no questions asked — to lower the fever. It might sound strange, but this is the first thing we would think of if someone was sweating and suffering from a high temperature. We recommend using unpasteurised, organic cider vinegar.

Important: If the patient is shivering this recipe is not appropriate, and you should seek medical advice.

– KARIN

THINGS YOU'LL NEED

500 ml (17 fl oz/2 cups) cool water

1–2 tablespoons vinegar

1 pair of long, woolly socks

1 or 2 towels

GET STARTED

The patient should be in bed, resting. Take a bowl, fill it with cool water and add the vinegar.

Soak the socks in this solution, wring them out slightly, keeping them nice and wet, and slide them over the feet and calves. Put a dry towel around the socks to prevent the bed from getting wet. After 45 minutes, if the patient's temperature hasn't gone down, replace the socks with freshly soaked socks.

Remove the socks if your patient's feet or hands are cold or if the patient starts shivering.

WHY WE BELIEVE IT WORKS

Vinegar stimulates the blood flow and has a fever-reducing effect. It also boosts the immune system and helps waste products to break down more quickly.

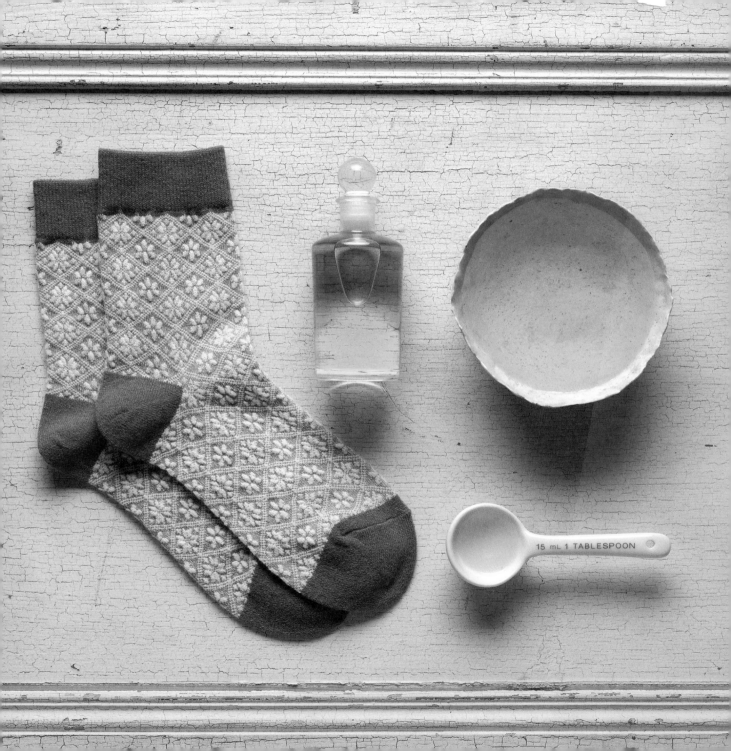

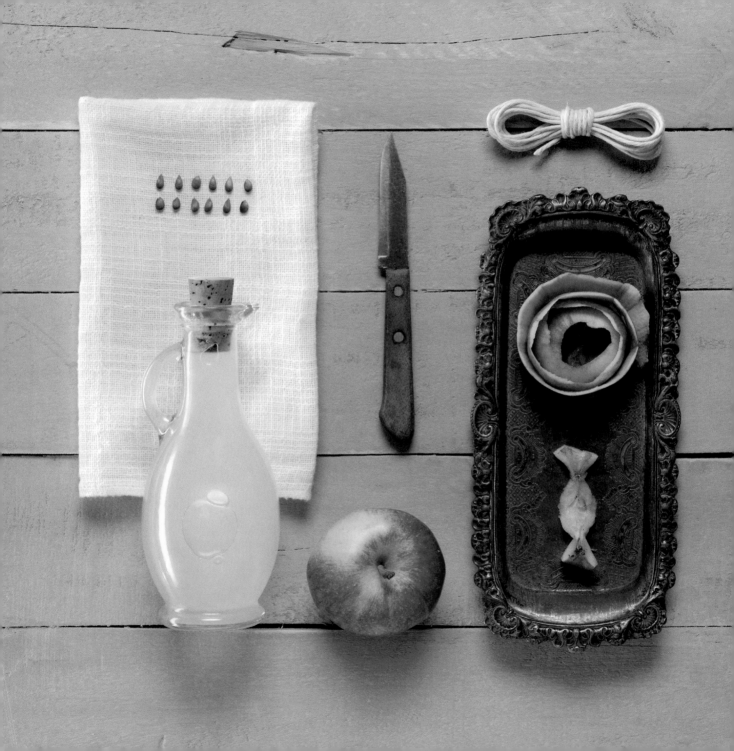

HOMEMADE APPLE CIDER VINEGAR

An all-rounder

It's possible to make vinegar from any fruit containing sugar, but apple cider vinegar is a favourite and is highly praised by Austrians for its healing benefits. The following recipe will give you a low acidity apple cider vinegar. The shelf life of vinegar is so long, that you might have consumed it, before it goes off.

– KARIN

THINGS YOU'LL NEED

2–3 apples, cut into small pieces (include peel and core)

2 × 1 litre (34 fl oz) wide-necked glass jars

approx. 600 ml (20 fl oz/2½ cups) water, at room temperature, enough to fill a jar

2 tablespoons honey

cheesecloth or fine muslin

piece of string, or a rubber band

GET STARTED

Place the apple chunks in a sterilized jar and add enough water to fill the jar. Stir in the honey. Cover the jar with a piece of cloth and secure it. Leave in a warm, dark, dry place.

After about two weeks, the water will become cloudy and a white foam will appear on the surface. Alcoholic fermentation is taking place as natural sugars change into alcohol. When the apple pieces sink to the bottom, strain the solution into a sterilized jar and cover with the cloth as before. Store the liquid for a further 4–6 weeks (light will slow or kill vinegar production).

The alcohol will now start to convert into acetic acid through acid fermentation and a white, gelatinous layer will form on the surface. This is called 'the mother of vinegar' and is made up of vinegar bacteria and cellulose – perfectly fine for consumption – which makes the vinegar more wholesome. Colour changes and cloudy deposits occur naturally in unpasteurized vinegar.

Start tasting your vinegar regularly after about 6 weeks. If an alcoholic smell remains, store the vinegar for a while longer and taste it periodically until there is no alchoholic flavour. Bottle the vinegar and seal it tightly with a non-corrosive lid for everyday use. You may separate the mother of vinegar from the vinegar solution and add it to unprocessed, unpasteurised, organic apple cider. This will accelerate the process for future stronger batches.

WHY WE BELIEVE IT WORKS

It is rich in natural enzymes and supports our natural bodily functions. It breaks up mucus, aids metabolism and increases the body's uptake of important minerals and nutrients from our food. It improves digestion and blood circulation. It is also anti-inflammatory, antibacterial, supports wound healing, prevents the spread of putrefactive bacteria in the gut, improves kidney performance and tightens tissue and skin. And it's a sublime hair conditioner!

HORSERADISH NECKLACE

Mum made this to treat fever and tonsillitis (and to make me look pretty!)

A horseradish necklace might sound strange, but it was quite normal in my home. Whenever I was in bed with fever and tonsillitis, Mum would make me a necklace of fresh horseradish slices. If I were feeling really poorly, I would get the fried onion treatment at the same time (see page 55). Onion halves would decorate the floor around my bed so my airways could be cleared by their antibacterial vapours.

– KARIN

THINGS YOU'LL NEED

fresh horseradish root

needle

piece of string

balm or ointment

soft muslin cloth

GET STARTED

Wash but don't peel the horseradish. Cut it into 3–5 mm (⅛–¼ in.) slices and place in tepid water to soak for 5 minutes. Using a needle and string, poke holes into the horseradish slices and thread the slices onto the string to make a necklace. Apply protective balm to your neck in the area where the horseradish will touch your skin. Put the necklace on and tie it at the back. Cover with a soft muslin to prevent the horseradish from drying out.

My mum recently reminded me that as soon as the necklace is dry, you must replace it with a fresh one. This is because the beneficial ingredients are only active when the horseradish is fresh and moist.

WHY WE BELIEVE IT WORKS

Horseradish lowers fever and is a traditional remedy for unblocking the airways. It has antibiotic and antiviral properties and contains flavonoids and vitamins C and B1.

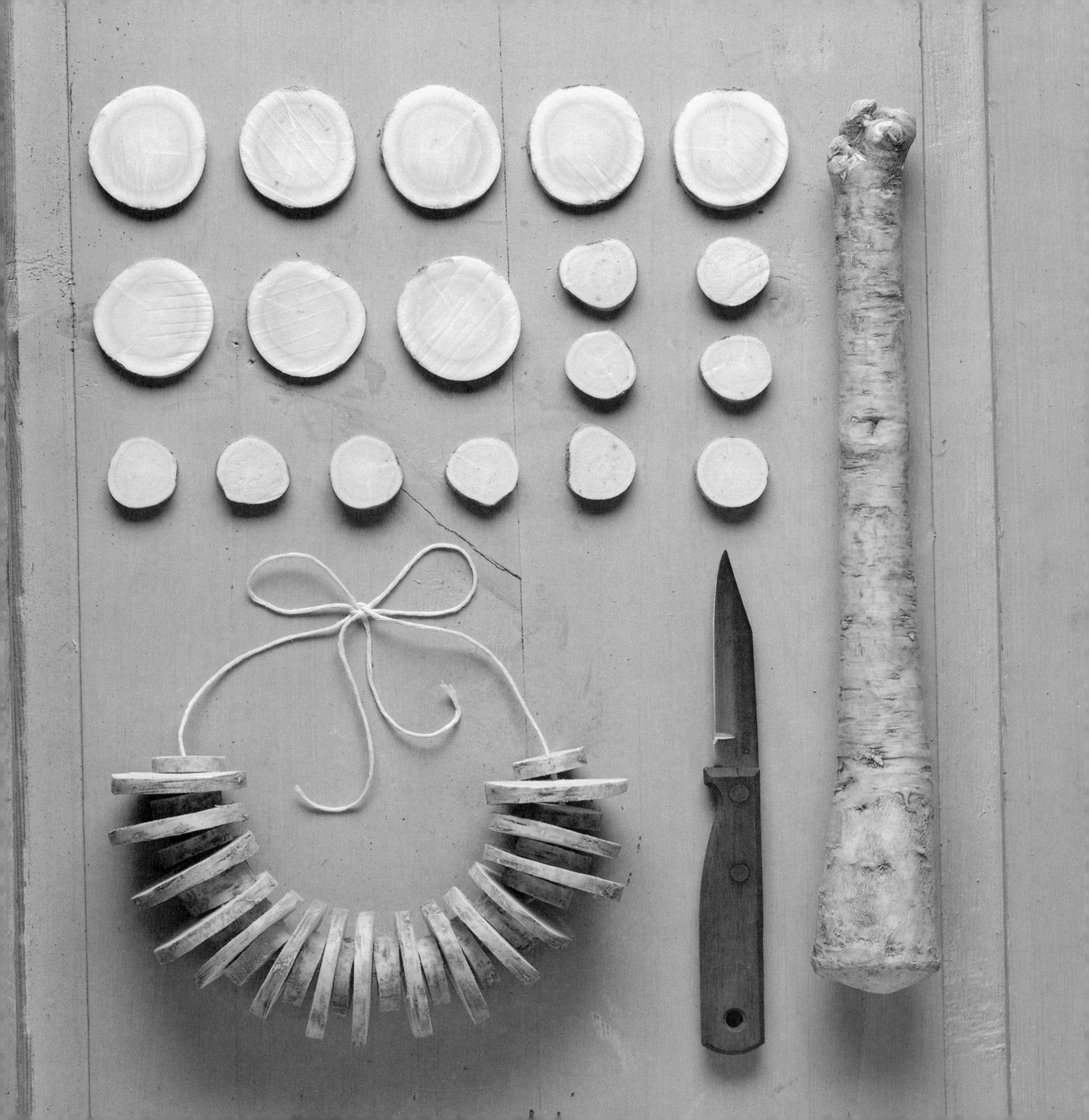

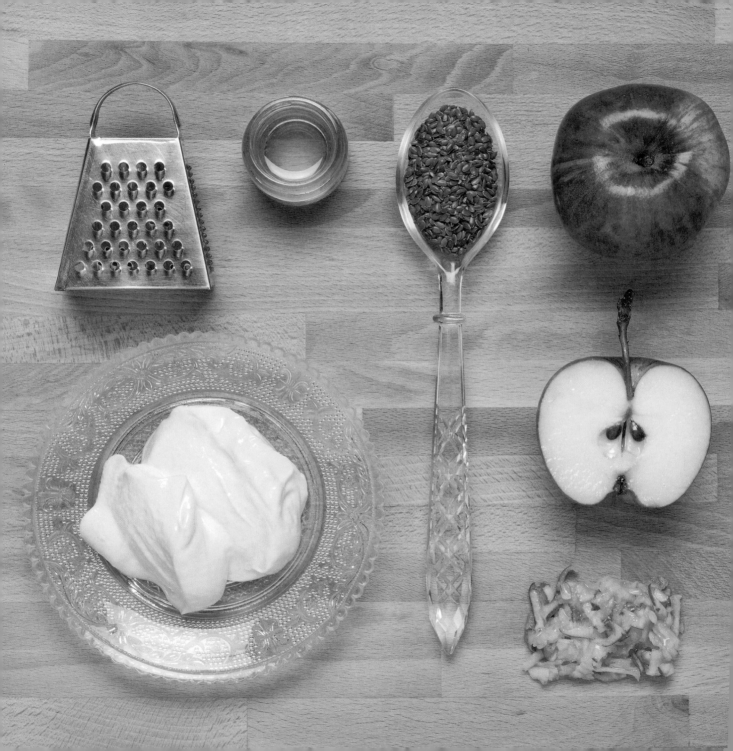

APPLE CURD

Consider this for constipation

THINGS YOU'LL NEED

125 g (4 oz/½ cup) curd cheese or quark

1 apple, grated

1 teaspoon linseeds (flaxseeds)

1 teaspoon honey

This tastes delicious and is very easy to make. If you want to eat this straight away, you'll need to soak the linseeds (also known as flaxseeds) overnight before adding them to the curd.

- KARIN

GET STARTED

Put the curd in a bowl and add the grated apple, linseeds and honey. Mix well. Add a little water to suit your personal taste.

If you haven't soaked the linseeds overnight, crush them and let the mixture rest for 10 minutes before eating. This gives the linseeds time to release all their beneficial properties.

WHY WE BELIEVE IT WORKS

When my sister did some research into the health benefits of apples, she decided that we simply must eat more of them. They have a high nutritional value, contain many vitamins and trace elements, and aid digestion. The fruit acids in apples inhibit harmful enzymes and putrefactive bacteria in the gut.

Curd is anti-inflammatory, sooths digestion and contains many minerals and vitamins. It will also boost your metabolism.

Linseeds are a food and a medicine in one. They aid digestion, protect the lining of the intestines and are rich in dietary fibre. They are also high in minerals and vitamins. Crush or soak them before eating.

Honey is a mild and natural laxative.

PREMIUM
LIP BALM

Try this for chapped lips

THINGS YOU'LL NEED

1 glass or ceramic bowl

15 g (½ oz) beeswax

15 g (½ oz) virgin, cold pressed
coconut oil

30 g (¾ oz) Jojoba oil

3 drops of honey

3 drops of lavender

8-9 small lip balm tubs

As if getting a cold isn't bad enough, now your smile
has been wiped off your lovely lips as they are cracked
and dry. But this will change in no time thanks to our
- not strictly Austrian - extremely nourishing lip balm,
made by you! (Be sure to stock up on organic bees wax
pellets in time.)

- NICI

GET STARTED

Mix all ingredients together, except for the lavender
oil, in a glass or ceramic bowl. On a low heat, melt the
ingredients carefully and slowly over steaming water. Be
careful not to overheat as the ingredients are extremely
heat sensitive. Once all the bees wax has liquefied, add
the lavender oil to the mixture whilst stirring. Now,
quickly and carefully, pour the liquid into the lip balm
jars. Beeswax hardens very fast when cooling.

WHY WE BELIEVE IT WORKS

Beeswax is a very agreeable fat component and can be
easily mixed with the other ingredients in this recipe.
It has skin protecting and moisturising properties and
a soothing effect.

Coconut oil is antibacterial, antiviral and fungicidal.
It fights infections, supports the skin's natural healing
process and reduces scar formation.

Jojoba oil has a natural sun protection factor of 3-4
and is rich in Vitamin A and E. It is easily absorbed
by the skin, penetrating the deepest layers. Although
it is called an oil, it is actually a liquid wax.

Honey is a natural antiseptic agent, is antibacterial
and anti-inflammatory. It facilitates in healing wounds.

Lavender oil is antiseptic, antibacterial, anti-fungal,
anti-inflammatory and has pain-relieving properties.

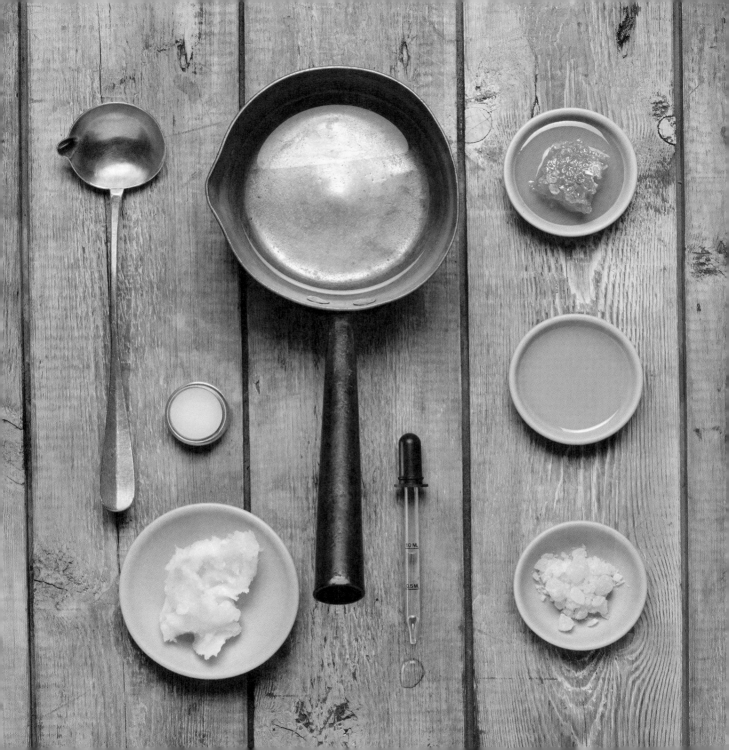

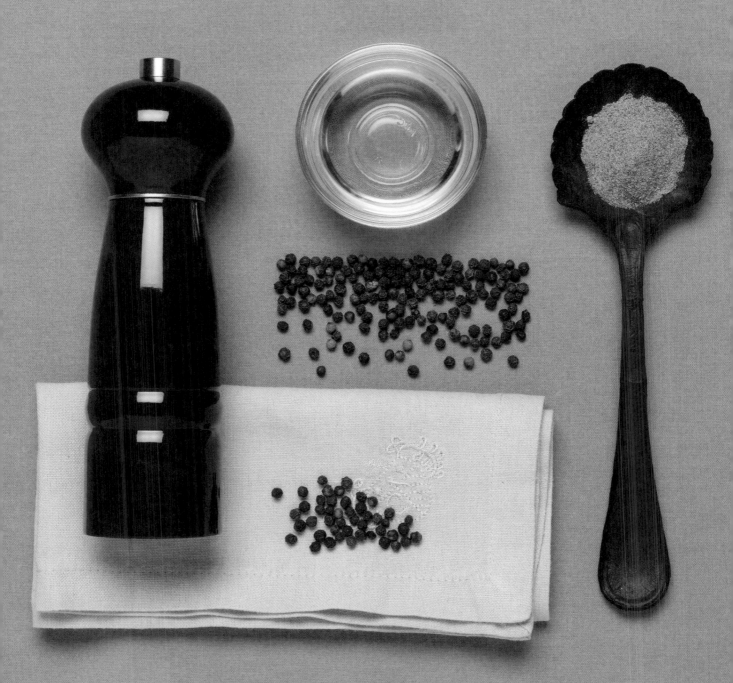

VINEGAR
& PEPPER
CLOTH

When we have the sniffles

THINGS YOU'LL NEED

small piece of linen or strong
paper tissue

homemade apple cider vinegar (page 13)

black pepper corns for grinding

Good old vinegar! It really is a superhero amongst
natural remedies — and now stars in this traditional
home remedy for a runny nose. Apple cider vinegar has
been used as a medicinal substance for 4,000 years and,
as we all know, an apple a day keeps the doctor away!
Ideally, use homemade apple cider vinegar or the best
organic cider vinegar you can find.

– NICI

GET STARTED

Take the piece of linen or tissue and dip it in the
vinegar until it's soaked. Grind the pepper over
the top.

Lie down on your back on a comfy sofa or cosy bed and
place the piece of linen or tissue (peppery side facing
up) on your bare chest for no longer than 20 minutes.
Breathe deeply!

For the best results, repeat this ritual several times
a day.

WHY WE BELIEVE IT WORKS

Black pepper stimulates circulation in your airways
and doubles as a decongestant.

Vinegar acts as a disinfectant and is antibacterial.

HERB POUCH

Said to prevent nightmares

THINGS YOU'LL NEED

3 teaspoons chamomile flowers

3 teaspoons peppermint

3 teaspoons rosemary

3 teaspoons sage

3 teaspoons valerian

3 teaspoons thyme

small piece of cotton fabric

piece of string

... not a single sheep!

If you toss and turn at night, are kept awake with thoughts about tomorrow's to-do list, or are troubled by bad dreams, this aromatic remedy may help prevent nightmares and lead to a lovely, floaty, restful sleep.

– NICI

GET STARTED

Place the ingredients in the centre of your piece of fabric and fold the corners in, so the herbs sit like the stuffing inside a cushion. Secure with string and place inside your pillowcase or next to it. Goodbye, Freddy Krueger!

WHY WE BELIEVE IT WORKS

Chamomile acts as a sedative and helps to relieve anxiety and insomnia.

Peppermint is antimicrobial and antispasmodic.

Rosemary is cleansing; sage contains antibacterial oils and can act as an antiperspirant; thyme calms the mind and relieves pain.

Valerian (the most important ingredient) is calming, relaxing and has a soporific effect.

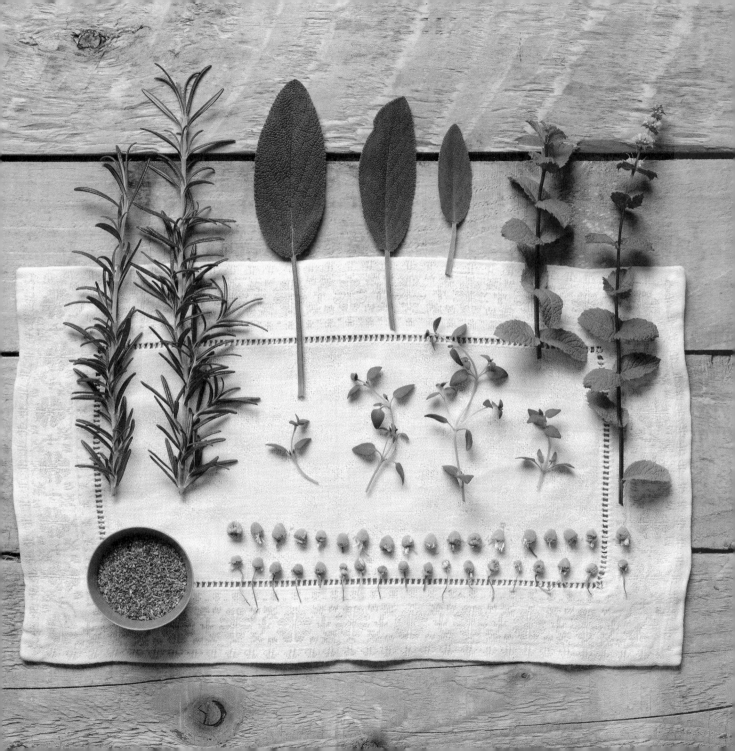

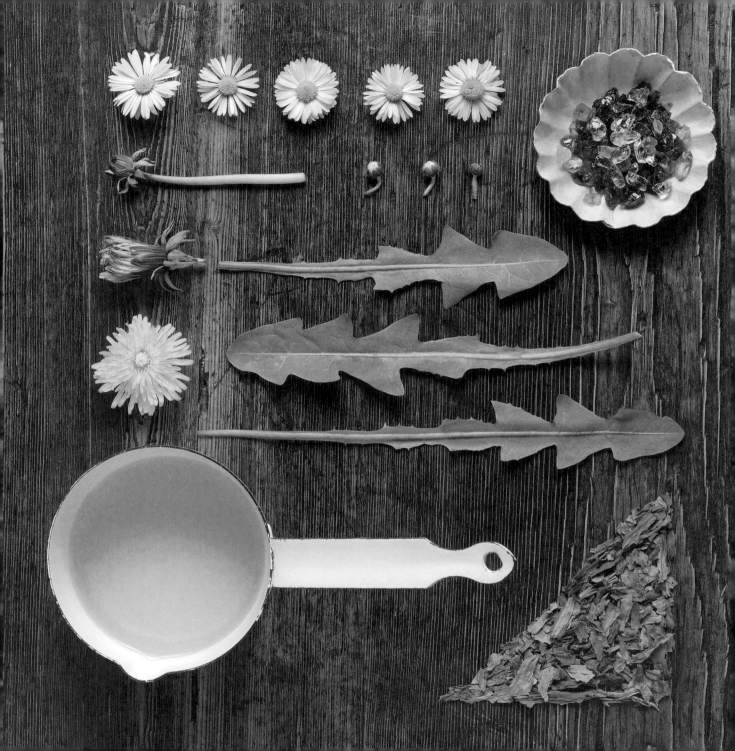

DANDELION DETOX SYRUP

Traditional detoxifier and
metabolism booster

THINGS YOU'LL NEED

50 g (2 oz) dandelion flowers
(remove all green bits)

50 g (2 oz) ribwort plantain leaves

50 g (2 oz) daisy flowers

1.2 litres (40 fl oz/5 cups) water

1 kg (2 lb 3 oz/5½ cups lightly packed)
brown sugar

2 × 1 litre (34 fl oz) wide-necked
glass jar

This is a great traditional Austrian recipe that has
been passed down through generations. Every plant you
need, grows in Austrian gardens or along mountain
trails: humble little flowers and herbs, just waiting to
be picked, ready to deliver their healing powers. This
syrup is popular in Austria as a blood purifier and for
detoxing.

– NICI

GET STARTED

Put the dandelion flowers, ribwort plantain leaves and
daisy flowers in a saucepan with the water and let them
soak for 2 hours.

Bring to the boil and then reduce the heat slightly.
Simmer gently to infuse for 30 minutes and then strain.

Return the liquid to the pan while it is still hot, add
the sugar and stir until it has completely dissolved. If
needed, return to the heat, stirring constantly, until
the liquid becomes syrupy.

Finally, pour into sterilized preserving jars and store
in a cool, dark place – it will stay fresh for up to 6–8
months. It tastes just lovely on some bread and butter
or as a sweetener in your tea.

We recommend 1 teaspoon a day.

WHY WE BELIEVE IT WORKS

Both dandelions and daisies are detoxifying. Dandelions
also stimulate the metabolism.

Ribwort plantain leaves are astringent, wound-healing
and blood-purifying.

HORSERADISH PARCEL

Try it for sinusitis and head colds

Make up this little parcel of relief whenever you have blocked sinuses or a numbing head cold.

– NICI

THINGS YOU'LL NEED

fresh horseradish root

small square of thin cotton cloth, such as muslin

piece of string

GET STARTED

Clean the horseradish and grate it as finely as possible (you'll need roughly 1 teaspoon). Place this on the centre of the piece of cloth and draw up the sides to cover it. Tie into a small parcel with the string.

Now place the horseradish parcel just above the nape of your neck, but don't leave it for longer than 3 minutes. Keep an eye on the time to avoid skin irritation.

WHY WE BELIEVE IT WORKS

Horseradish loosens phlegm, is antimicrobial and encourages blood flow. It could be exactly what you need!

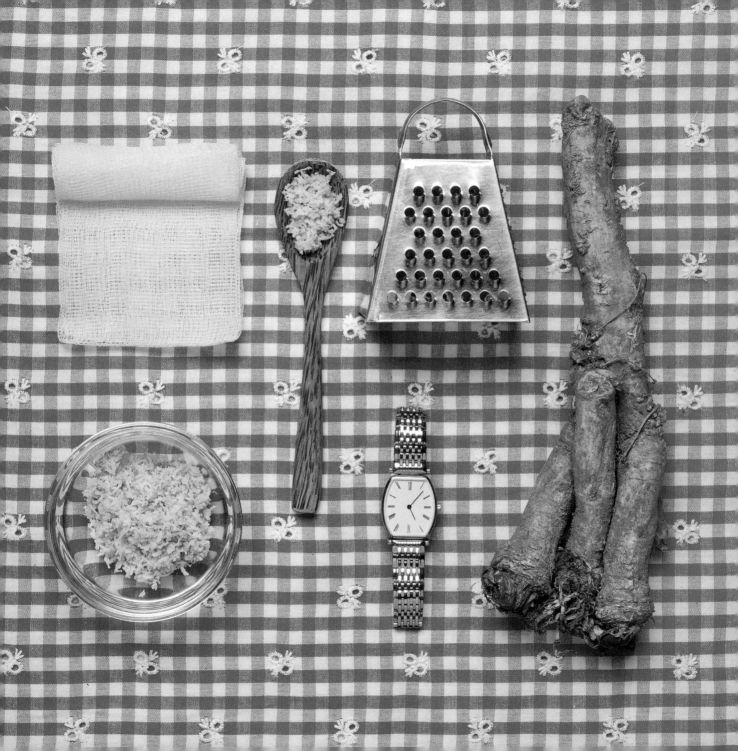

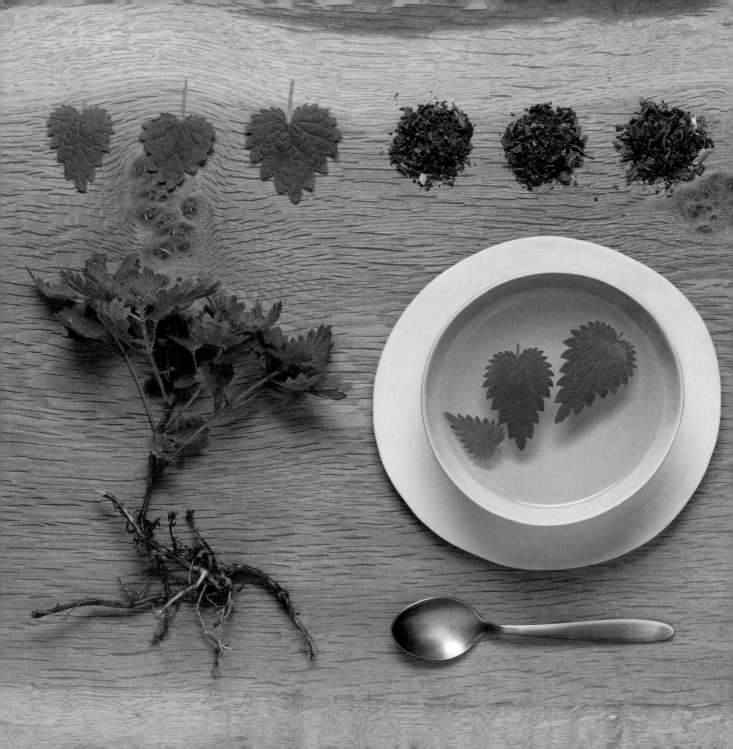

NETTLE TEA

Mum's recipe to cleanse the blood and Grandad's answer to many other things

Nettles are one of my favourite plants. This surprisingly delicious infusion is easy to make. You'll need to pick the nettle leaves or dig up the roots before the plant produces flowers. The beneficial properties of nettles leaves are most potent before it flowers. Try to find nettles in the woods or in areas far away from roads. I would advise using gloves, although my mum has picked fresh nettles with her bare hands for as long as I can remember. She says the stings help prevent rheumatism! Nici's grandad jumps naked into a bed of nettles sometimes as often as once a week, to benefit from their healing properties.

Wash the nettles and use them right away or dry them and store in a jar until needed. If you want to use them in cooking, take a rolling pin and roll over the nettles a few times to break the stinging hairs. Once you've done this, the nettles are totally edible and can be used to make delicious salads and soups.

– KARIN

THINGS YOU'LL NEED

dried or freshly picked young nettle leaves or roots (if you're using roots, be sure to wash off all the soil)

250 ml (8½ fl oz/1 cup) water

1 teaspoon nettle leaves (3–4 leaves)

GET STARTED

Put 1 teaspoon nettle leaves in a cup and add boiling water. Leave to infuse for 10 minutes, then strain and drink immediately.

For nettle roots, put a handful of them in a pot, cover with 1 litre of water and bring to a boil. Remove from the heat immediately and leave for a couple of hours before straining and drinking.

WHY WE BELIEVE IT WORKS

Nettles are nutritious, anti-allergenic, antispasmodic, blood-cleansing, blood-building, high in vitamin C and iron, have antihistamine properties, and have been used in the treatment of diabetes and eczema. Nettles can also be helpful in relieving the pain of arthritis.

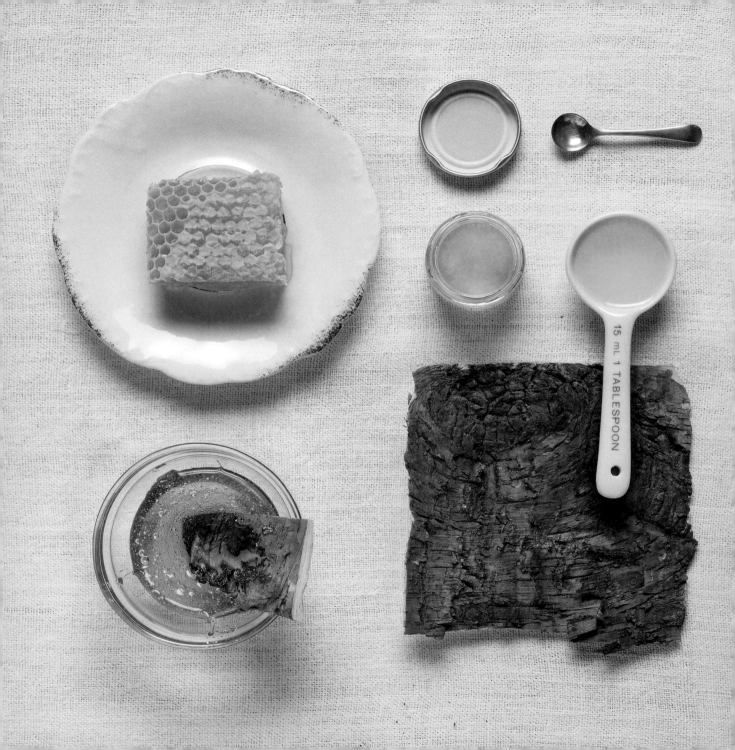

SAP
OINTMENT

A soothing all-rounder

Tree huggers have known it for a long time: hugging
a tree once in a while makes everything better,
especially if your choice of tree is an Austrian larch,
as their sap is full of healing power. This *Pechsalbe*
(sap ointment) helps your skin to heal, can be used
to sooth varicose veins, calms rheumatism and will
eliminate the odd clavus.

– NICI

THINGS YOU'LL NEED

30 g (1 oz) larch sap
(available from online health shops)

75 ml (2½ fl oz) olive oil

20 g (¾ oz) beeswax

small container

GET STARTED

Heat the sap, olive oil and beeswax in a small pan and
mix well until the sap is fully dissolved.

Now pour your ointment into a small, clean container
and wait for it to cool down. If you keep the container
closed and stored in a cool and dry place, this very
useful ointment will stay fresh for up to 18 months.

WHY WE BELIEVE IT WORKS

Just as sap seals the wounds in tree bark, it also helps
human skin to heal. In combination with olive oil, which
contains antioxidants, vitamin E, and beeswax, which is
antibiotic, larch sap is known to prevent infection,
soothe insect bites and corns, and even provide relief
for rheumatism and blisters.

CURD WRAP

My mum used it when I
had tonsillitis

I admit, this will be messy to make and you will smell
like an Austrian dessert, but you're ill with tonsillitis,
and desperate times call for desperate measures! On the
bright side, this recipe is the superhero of all curd
recipes and could sort out your sore throat in no time.
My favourite.

- NICI

THINGS YOU'LL NEED

1 tea towel (dish cloth)

250–500 g (8½–17 oz) curd cheese
or *Topfen*

safety pin

large towel

GET STARTED

Fold the tea towel into a long strip. Place around
100 g (3½ oz) of curd in a line along the strip.

Carefully wrap the towel with curd around your neck
so that the curd touches the skin. Secure with a small
safety pin.

It is a good idea to wrap another (large) towel around
your neck, because, like I said, this is a messy affair.

Now have a little nap. Maybe you'll have a dream about
Topfenstrudel, a delicious Austrian dessert!

As soon as the curd has dried, repeat up to three times.

WHY WE BELIEVE IT WORKS

Curd has anti-inflammatory qualities, soothes pains
and is cooling. When curd comes into contact with the
skin, it produces lactic acid which opens the pores and
stimulates blood flow. As the body heat warms the curd,
it absorbs inflammation and loosens phlegm.

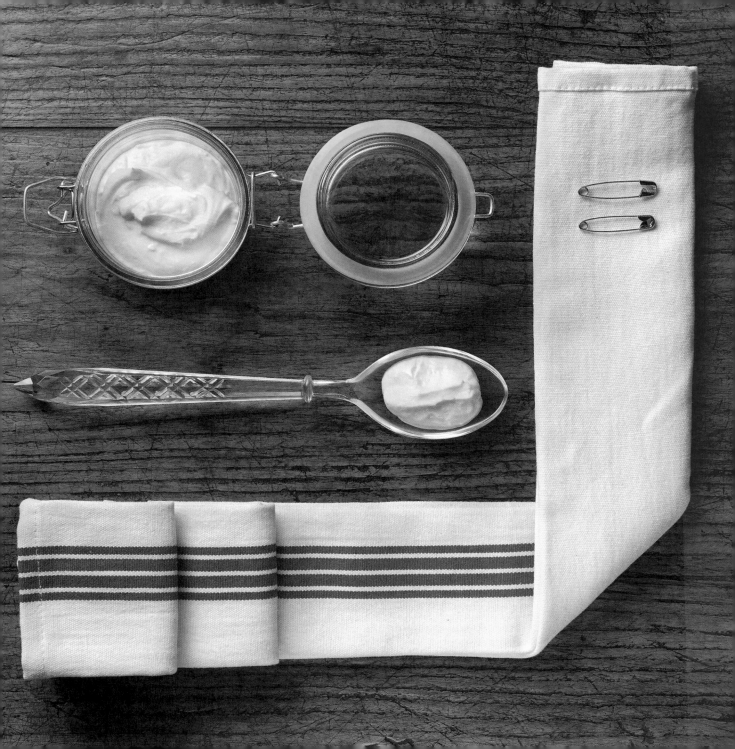

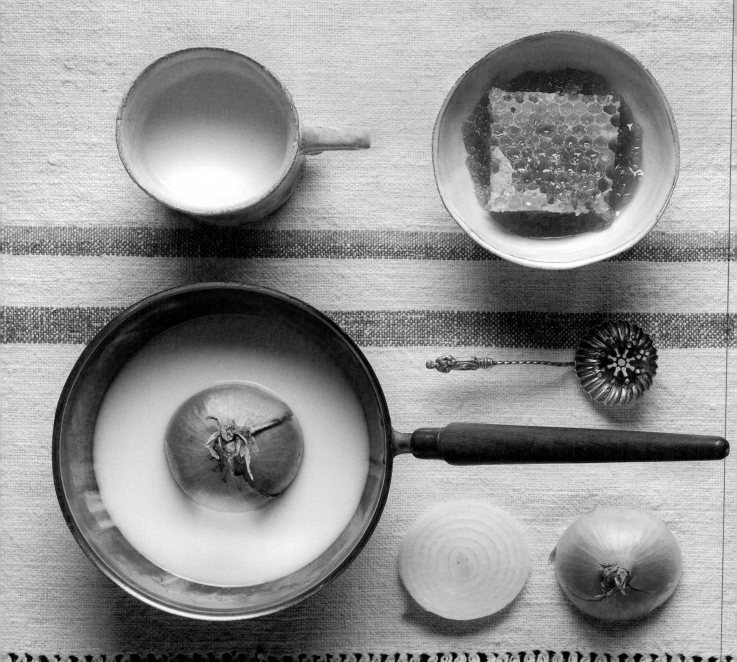

HOT
ONION
MILK

My mum's answer to coughs

THINGS YOU'LL NEED

500 ml (17 fl oz/2 cups) milk

2 large onions, diced

1–2 teaspoons honey per cup

You will probably find all the ingredients for this very simple recipe in your home without having to pop to the shops. How convenient!

– KARIN

GET STARTED

Heat the milk in a saucepan to a gentle simmer then add the onions. (Use almond milk, soya milk or water if you don't like the idea of using cow's milk.)

Remove from the heat immediately and leave to infuse for 20 minutes.

Strain into a cup or mug. Add the honey and drink the mixture to soothe your cough. Please make sure that you only add the honey just before drinking the milk, as honey is sensitive to heat.

If you don't drink all the onion milk at once, you can reheat the remainder gently in a saucepan.

WHY WE BELIEVE IT WORKS

Onions loosen phlegm and have antibacterial as well as anti-inflammatory properties, amongst many others.

Honey has been prized for thousands of years for its healing properties. It strengthens your immune system, prevents bacterial growth and reduces fever. It is also antispasmodic or anticonvulsant, and mucus-dissolving.

GRANDMA'S SECRET

When I had bronchitis

THINGS YOU'LL NEED

150 g (5 oz) quince

250 ml (8½ fl oz/1 cup) water

grated zest of 1 unwaxed lemon

honey, to taste

rye bread

Grandma's recipes are usually the best. This one is a real treat, because as well as being effective, it also tastes absolutely yummy.

- NICI

GET STARTED

Peel the quince, cut into small cubes and place into a saucepan. Pour the water over the cubes and bring to the boil. Reduce the heat and simmer gently until tender.

Next, push the quince through a sieve into a bowl. Add the lemon zest and plenty of honey to the puréed quince and stir.

Toast some rye bread (in true Granny style) and spread the quince over the top. *Guten Appetit*!

WHY WE BELIEVE IT WORKS

Quince is a good source of vitamin C, iodine and zinc. It is also rich in mucilage, which forms a protective layer over inflamed mucous membranes and is healing to the airwaves.

Honey has invigorating and antibacterial qualities.

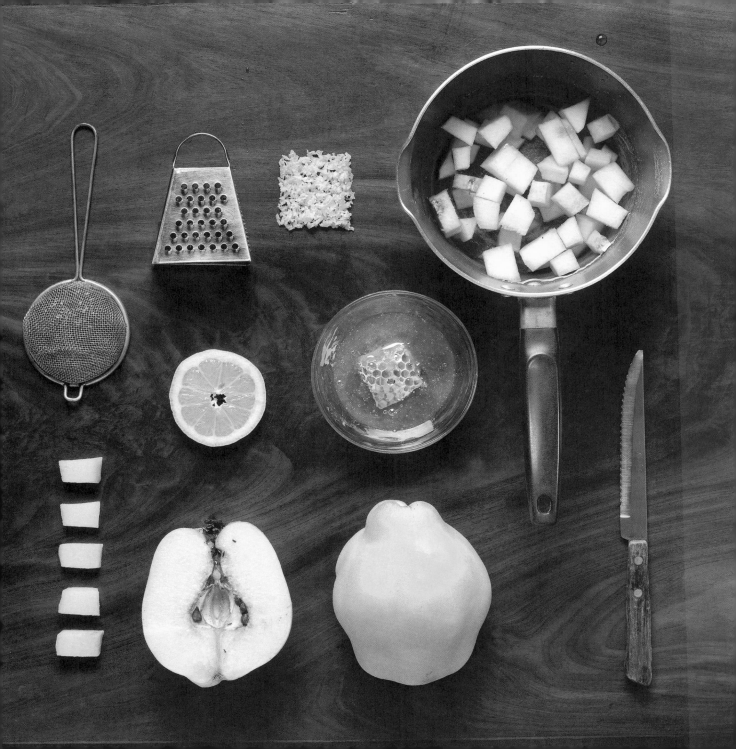

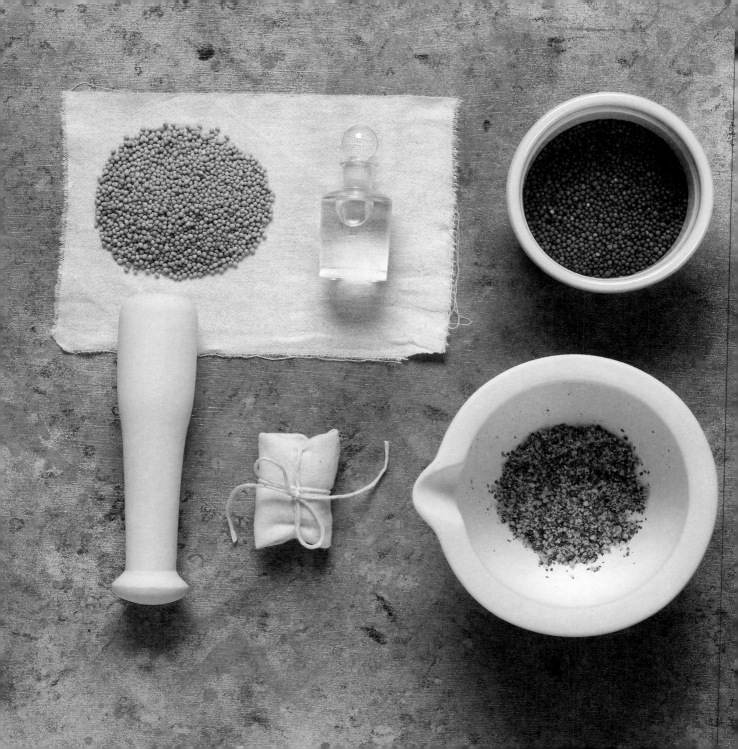

MUSTARD
SEED
COMPRESS

When my sister had sinusitis

This remedy involves using a pestle and mortar,
so you're allowed to feel incredibly professional —
crushing seeds and all — like a proper pharmacist!

– NICI

THINGS YOU'LL NEED

2 tablespoons mustard seeds
(brown and/or yellow)

pestle and mortar

1 tablespoon warm water

small linen cloth

piece of string

GET STARTED

Crush the mustard seeds in the pestle and mortar. Mix
with the warm water to form a paste. Spread the mustard
paste over the centre of the linen cloth, fold the edges
in to seal the paste inside and secure with string.

Press the little mustard parcel against your cheeks and
forehead, remove after 5-10 minutes. It's a good idea to
check inbetween, as the sensitive skin on your face can
become irritated.

Wash your face with warm water after the treatment. Be
very careful here: mustard seeds irritate the mucous
membranes, so take care the paste does not get into your
eyes. (But if it does, worry not: simply rinse well with
plenty of clean water.)

WHY WE BELIEVE IT WORKS

Mustard seeds are disinfecting, anticonvulsive and can
be used to treat inflammation, rheumatism and headaches.

CHAMOMILE & SALT INHALATION

This relieved my symptoms of a cold and cleared my airways

THINGS YOU'LL NEED

1 litre (34 fl oz/4 cups) water

handful of dried chamomile flowers

3 tablespoons sea salt

large towel

If you have a cold so bad you can't even breathe, we have the cure — just steam away the heavy head and blocked and swollen sinuses. And if that is not enough, this little gem of a remedy will also purify your skin and open your pores. We love side effects that make our skin look the most glorious, even when a head cold tries to ruin the day!

– NICI

GET STARTED

Bring the water to the boil in a saucepan, then remove from the heat. Add the chamomile flowers and sea salt.

Hold your head, face down, over the pan, about 20 cm (8 in.) away from the water, and cover your head with a large towel. Being careful to keep the towel away from the heat source. I always leave a small gap between the pan and my towel at first to allow my face to get used to the heat.

Inhale for 10 minutes and go to bed immediately after your treatment.

WHY WE BELIEVE IT WORKS

Chamomile disinfects, is antispasmodic and also has anti-inflammatory properties.

Sea salt loosens phlegm, strengthens your immune system, and acts as a disinfectant.

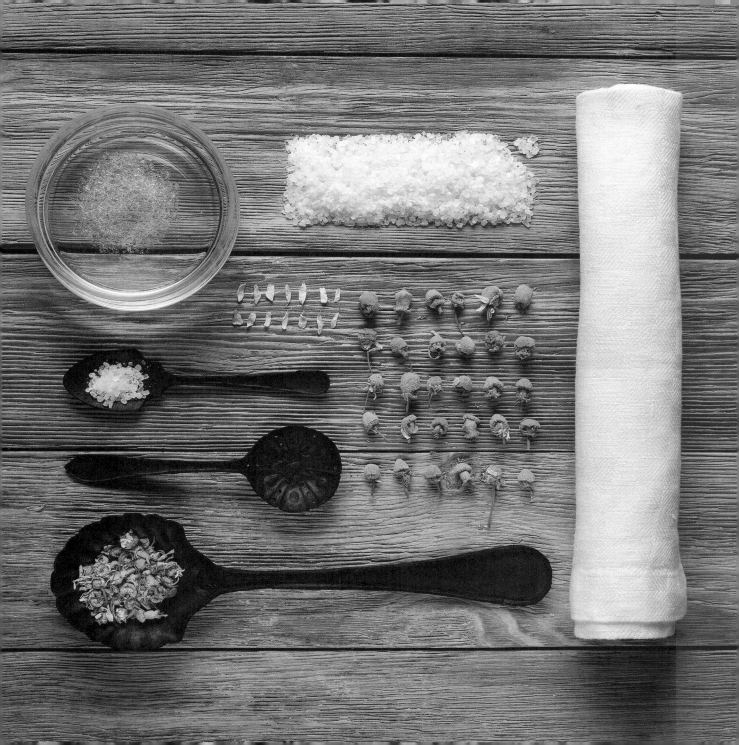

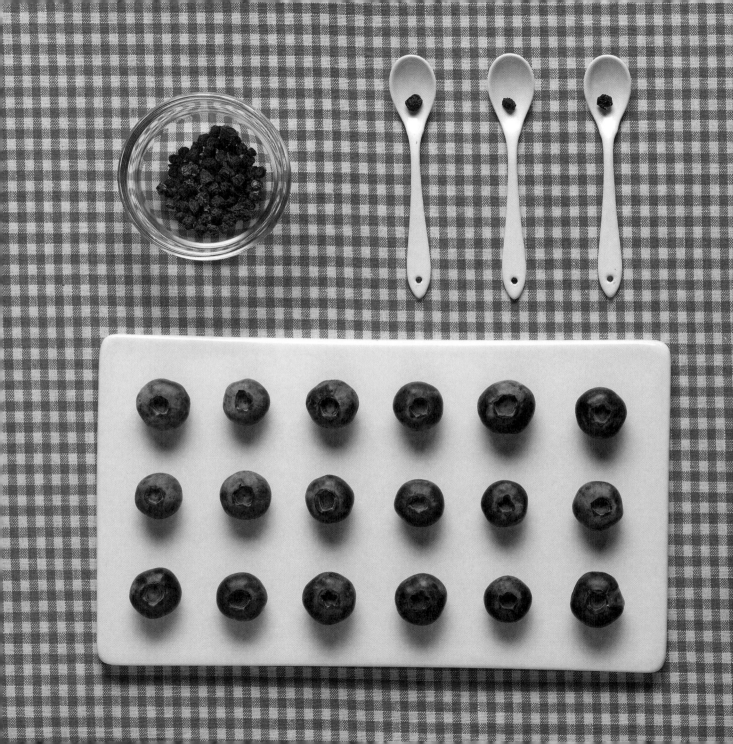

DRIED BLUEBERRY INFUSION

My nan's trick to treat diarrhoea

THINGS YOU'LL NEED

2-3 teaspoons dried blueberries (only use dried blueberries, as fresh ones have the opposite effect.)

250 ml (8½ fl oz/1 cup) water

As this might be a matter of urgency, here's the short version of an old remedy to settle your stomach and help alleviate diarrhoea: eat dried blueberries. There you go. Job done! This lovely tea is an equally effective, but slightly more elaborate version of this remedy.

– NICI

GET STARTED

Put the dried blueberries in a small saucepan and add the water. Bring to the boil, reduce the heat slightly and simmer for 10 minutes. Strain and drink throughout the day.

WHY WE BELIEVE IT WORKS

Dried blueberries have been known as an effective cure for diarrhoea since the Middle Ages. Both the berries and their leaves contain tannins which have an astringent effect.

FLOWERPOWER BREW

Family remedy to treat bronchitis

THINGS YOU'LL NEED

petals from 1 peony

250 g (9 oz/1 cup) crystallised sugar
(brown rock candy)

125 ml (4½ fl oz/½ cup) water

honey, to taste

Pray for a bunch of peonies from a visitor to your
sickbed — not because they will look lovely in a vase,
but because if you pluck 'em and cook 'em, they will
cure your ever-so-stubborn bronchitis. Only use peonies
that haven't been sprayed with pesticides.

- NICI

GET STARTED

Place the peony petals in a saucepan with the sugar and
water. Bring to the boil, reduce the heat and simmer for
10 minutes until the sugar is fully dissolved. Allow it
to cool and then add honey.

Take 1 tablespoon of this brew three times a day.

WHY WE BELIEVE IT WORKS

Due to their antispasmodic qualities, peonies have been
used for centuries by people across the world (including
our Austrian grandmothers) to treat an array of illnesses
from cramps to respiratory track infections and even
gynaecological problems.

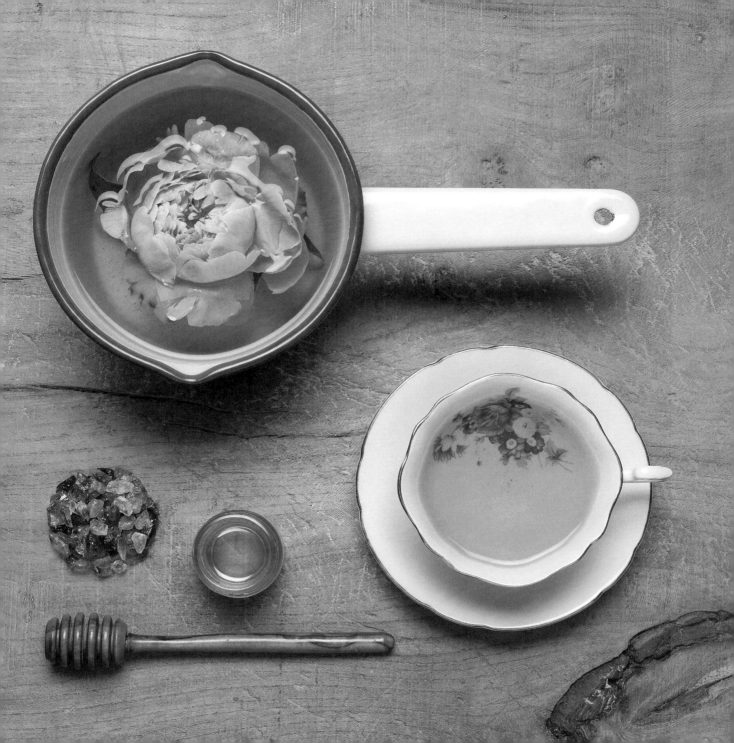

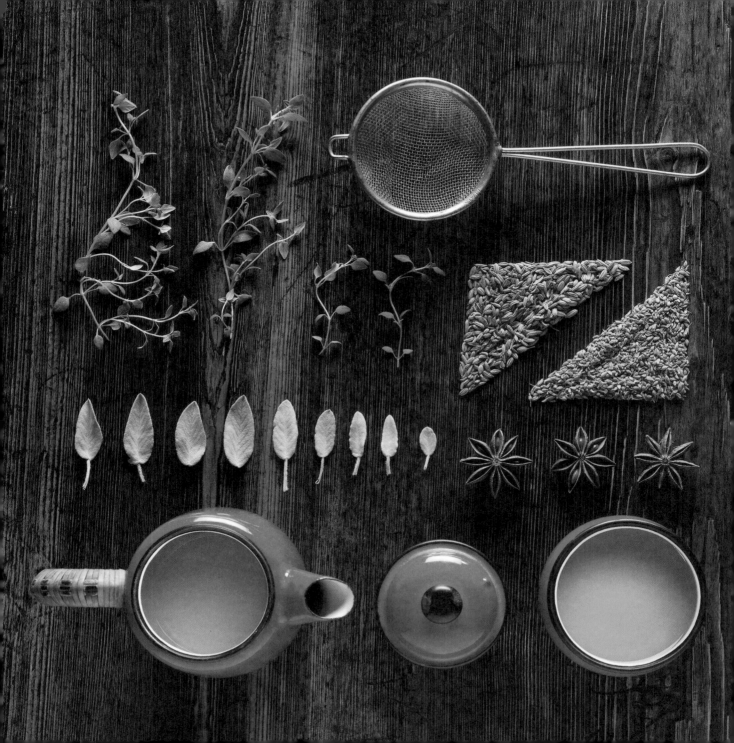

ANISEED, FENNEL & SAGE TEA

Try this for sinusitis

THINGS YOU'LL NEED

60 g (2 oz) aniseeds or
Chinese star anise

30 g (1 oz) fennel seeds

30 g (1 oz) sage leaves

40 g (1½ oz) thyme leaves

250 ml (8½ fl oz/1 cup) water,
per cup of tea

I love tea. English tea is the answer to a lot of little
niggles, especially: how will I ever get out of bed
in the morning? It is also a socially accepted first
response for all kind of bad news – a great all-rounder!
The one thing it's not good for, though, is to alleviate
sinusitis. For that you'll need a different kind of tea
such as this fresh-tasting infusion.

– NICI

GET STARTED

Mix the seeds and herbs together.

Use 1 generous teaspoon of this blend per cup. Boil
the water and pour into the cup. Infuse for 10 minutes,
then strain.

Drink 2 cups per day until the symptoms of sinusitis
go away.

Store the dried mixture in a cool, dry place.

WHY WE BELIEVE IT WORKS

Aniseeds and star anis are antibacterial, gently
anticonvulsant and contain essential oils. Their
cleansing tendencies have a beneficial effect on many
chronic illnesses.

Fennel seeds help to loosen phlegm. They also have
antiseptic properties.

Thyme acts as an antibacterial and disinfectant.
It's also anti-inflammatory.

Sage is fungicidal with antibacterial properties.

SPRUCE NEEDLE BATH

Try this for head colds, runny noses and coughs

If you feel a cold coming on, have a bath with this spruce tree essence. By the time you have filled the bath with water, the essence will not just be ready for your bath, but also smell like a lovely spruce forest.

– KARIN

THINGS YOU'LL NEED

3 fresh twigs from a spruce tree, washed

1 litre (34 fl oz/4 cups) water

GET STARTED

Cut the spruce twigs into small pieces, place them in a saucepan and add the water. Bring to the boil, reduce the heat to low, and simmer for 10 minutes.

Now remove the pan from the heat, cover with a cloth, and let the solution of twigs infuse for another 10 minutes while you run your bath.

Strain and add the solution to your bath. Relax in the bath for 20 minutes, breathing in deeply and taking in all the wonderful forest scents.

Go to bed immediately and rest.

WHY WE BELIEVE IT WORKS

Spruce needles have an invigorating and antispasmodic effect and stimulate the blood flow. The essential oils clear and disinfect the lungs and airways.

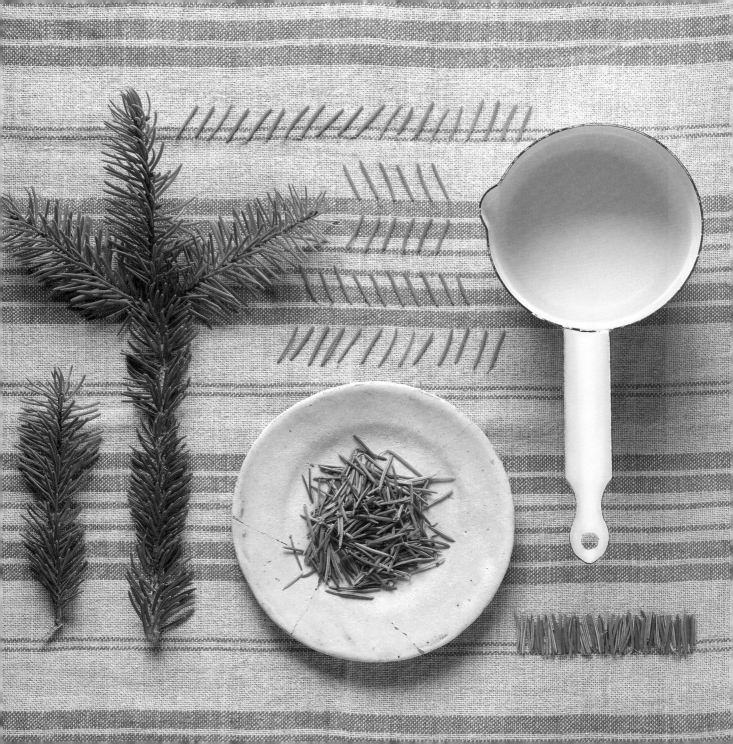

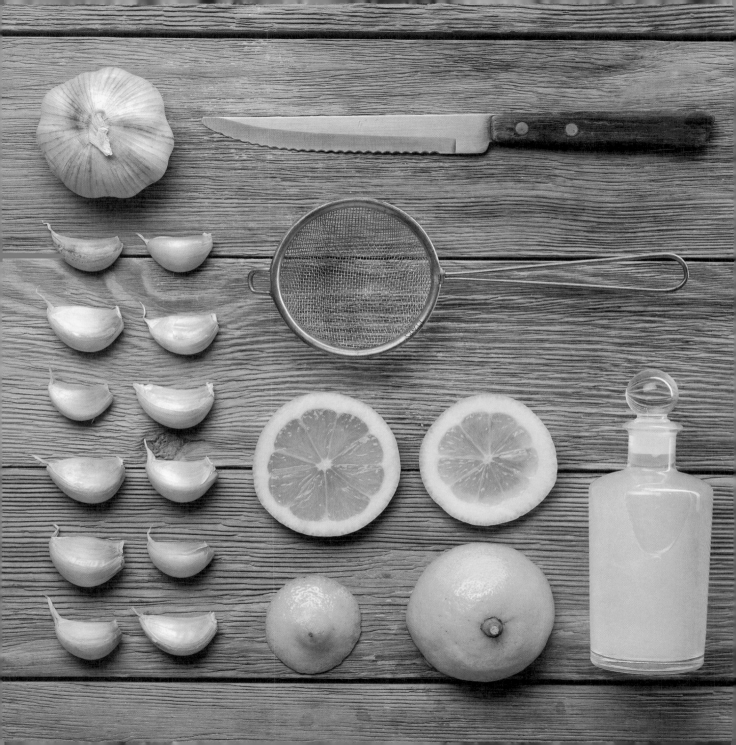

LEMON & GARLIC BREW

For sore throats and for boosting your immune system

THINGS YOU'LL NEED

½ unwaxed organic lemon

2 garlic cloves

120 ml (4 fl oz) water

Though this mixture is powerful and potent, it has a surprisingly low score on the smelliness scale. Be as brave as the Austrians and enjoy this recipe raw. Don't worry, it doesn't taste as scary as it sounds. In fact, it is quite pleasant. This recipe makes enough for about 1–2 people.

– KARIN

GET STARTED

Wash and peel the lemon thoroughly and cut it into small pieces.

Peel and chop the garlic. Combine the ingredients in a high-speed blender and blitz until smooth.

Enjoy 1–2 shots straight away and share the rest with your family. Drink 1–2 shots twice a day.

For best results, always consume this remedy when it's fresh and make small amounts if nobody else wants to share this miracle remedy with you.

Important: If you are the proud owner of a lemon tree or know of one that hasn't been sprayed with pesticides, then add the lemon peel to the blender too. Many nutrients are within the skin.

WHY WE BELIEVE IT WORKS

Garlic's antibacterial power was first scientifically proven in 1858 by the world famous microbiologist Louis Pasteur. The wonder drug has natural antibiotic properties, is rich in antioxidants and strengthens the immune system.

Lemons are antibacterial, antiseptic and antiviral, rich in vitamin C, calcium, potassium, magnesium, antioxidants and flavonoids. The peel contains vitamin C, calcium, potassium and flavonoids.

LAVENDER BATH

How we bathe away our stress
and tensions

I am still so surprised by how simple it is to make
this soothing bath essence. It's easiest to measure the
lavender flowers using a large teacup, as they weigh
practically nothing, and we don't need to be really
precise here. It's a simple 2:1 ratio, so for every one
teacup of flowers, simply use two teacups of water.

– KARIN

THINGS YOU'LL NEED

1 large teacup of dried or fresh
lavender flowers

2 large teacups water

GET STARTED

Whilst your bath is filling up, place the lavender
flowers in a pot. Put on the kettle, then pour the
boiling water over the lavender flowers and leave to
infuse for 10 minutes.

Strain, then add the solution to the warm bath water.
Stay in the bath no longer than 15 minutes, then go to
bed immediately afterwards and rest.

WHY WE BELIEVE IT WORKS

Lavender contains many essential oils, some of which
are relaxing and soothing. Warm water helps your skin
absorb these oils and they can be inhaled from steam
too. Lavender also has anti-inflammatory and antiseptic
properties which can help to heal wounds. The botanical
name for the plant, Lavandula, may be derived from the
Latin word *lavare* which means 'to wash'.

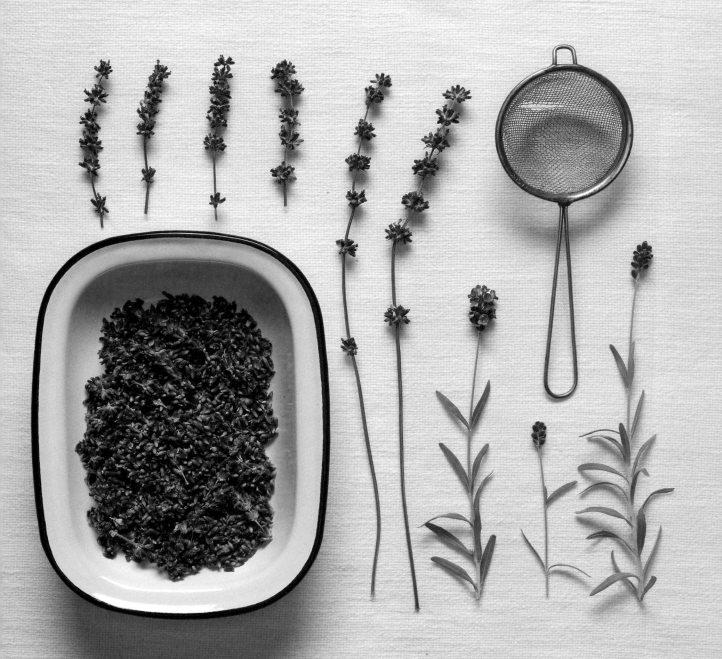

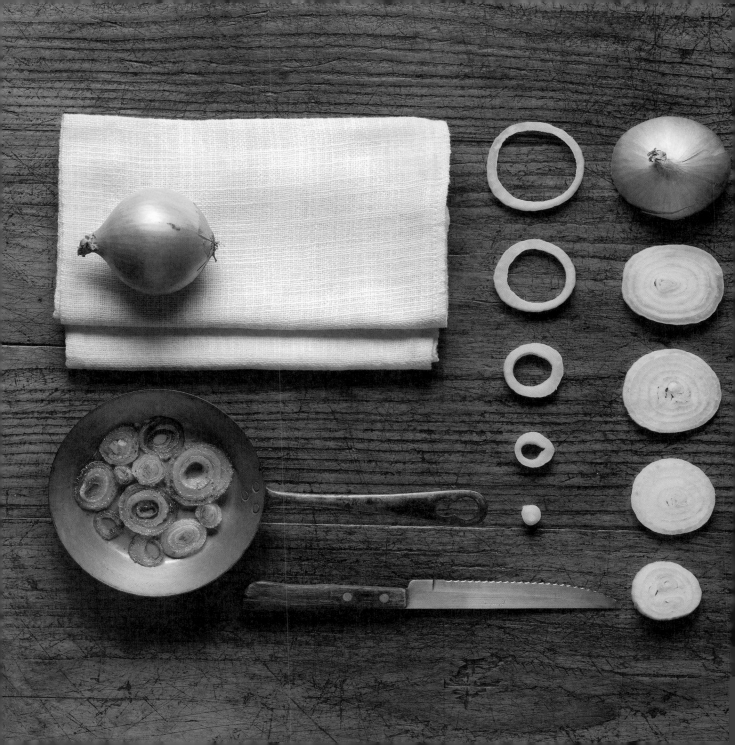

FRIED
ONION
WRAP

Mum used this for colds,
bronchitis and sore throats

This recipe is one of my mum's favourites, or at least I had that impression as a child. At the first sign of a severe cold or cough, she would announce that onions were the answer. Granted, you will end up smelling of fried onions, but this cure involves no preservatives or scary side-effects. My mum used finely woven muslin cloth to wrap the onions in, before tying them in place around me. This allowed the juices to seep into my skin whilst the onion vapours soothed my airways.

– KARIN

THINGS YOU'LL NEED

a little oil

1–2 onions, finely sliced

1 piece of cloth about the size of a dish cloth; preferably a natural fabric such as cotton muslin

1 piece of cloth or a towel, long enough to fit around the patient; again, preferably a natural fabric

GET STARTED

Heat the oil – you only need a tiny amount – in a frying pan and add the onions. Fry gently until soft and golden. (Austrians usually use lard to fry the onions for this recipe.)

Remove the onions from the pan whilst hot and spread them over the top half of the first piece of cloth. Fold the bottom half over the onions. Fold the ends of the cloth to enclose the onions. This will not be completely leak-proof and will allow the juices to seep through to the skin. The onions should now have cooled down slightly to safely place the parcel on your chest.

Wrap the second piece of cloth or towel around the upper body to keep the onions in place. This will soak up any of the oil if it leaks. Wrap a longer towel around your chest to keep everything in placé.

WHY WE BELIEVE IT WORKS

Onions are antibacterial, anti-inflammatory and disinfecting. They are also rich in Vitamins A, B1, C and E, all of which are powerful antioxidants.

BLACK MOOLI COUGH SYRUP

Mum's cough syrup

This recipe is not difficult at all but it is slightly challenging. It requires a bit of patience as well as some carving skills. The taste will remind you a little of conventional cough syrups. It is number two on my list of memorable home remedies, after Vinegar Socks (see page 10).

– KARIN

THINGS YOU'LL NEED

1 black mooli (daikon radish)

crystallised brown sugar (rock candy)

GET STARTED

Cut a lid off the mooli and scoop out one-third of the flesh from the middle, leaving a shell of about 1 cm (½ in.) width. Make a small hole at the bottom of the mooli with a skewer, so that the juices can seep through. Fill the mooli with crystallised brown sugar, cover with the mooli lid and place the mooli over a glass to collect the juices.

Make sure there is enough space in the glass for the juices to collect as you leave it overnight. As the sugar dissolves, it will extract the juices from the mooli, and drip into the glass below.

The resulting cough syrup can be safely stored in a covered jar in the fridge for a couple of days. Take 1 tablespoon three times a day to loosen phlegm.

WHY WE BELIEVE IT WORKS

Black mooli is bursting with healing minerals and vitamins. It has antimicrobial and antiviral properties and strengthens the immune system.

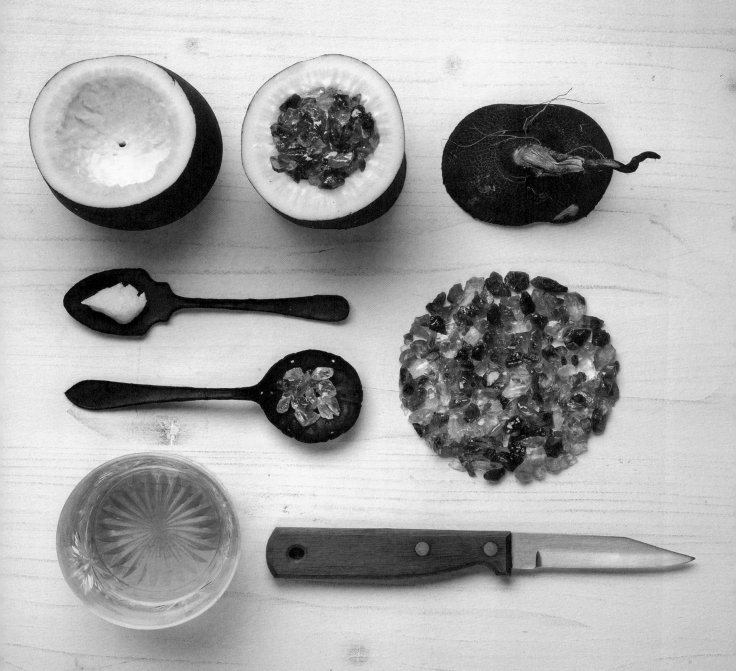

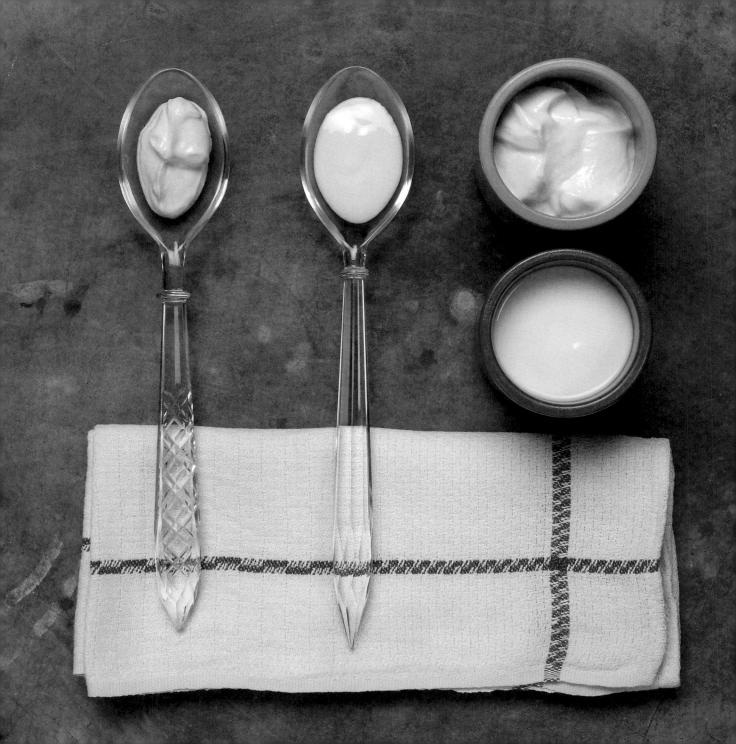

CURD PACK

My favourite sunburn remedy

Curd cheese (or *Topfen*) isn't just the Austrian super weapon for all kinds of illnesses, but it's also the main ingredient in a delicious *Topfenstrudel*, the lesser-known alternative to our famous *Apfelstrudel*. For this remedy, though, you'll need to divert the curd away from your mouth, so you can focus its healing powers on your burning skin. With its cooling and pain-relieving qualities, the good old curd pack has been successful in treating sunburn during many hot Austrian summers.

Important: A curd pack should not be used on broken skin.

– NICI

THINGS YOU'LL NEED

250 g (8½ oz/1 cup) curd cheese or *Topfen*

200 ml (7 fl oz/¾ cup) buttermilk

linen or cotton cloth or tea towel (dish cloth)

GET STARTED

Mix 3 tablespoons of curd with 2 tablespoons of buttermilk. Spread the mixture over a linen cloth or tea towel. Place the curd mix directly on the sunburnt skin and leave for 20–30 minutes. As soon as you notice the curd getting warmer or dry, replace with a new pack.

WHY WE BELIEVE IT WORKS

Both curd and buttermilk have anti-inflammatory properties and are understood to be healing and cooling.

SAGE TEA

Brew this for sore throat
and croakiness

Sage infusions are very effective in treating mouth,
throat and gum inflammation due to symptoms of a cold.
If you've never tried a sage infusion, you will love
this. It soothes your throat and tastes wonderful.

– KARIN

THINGS YOU'LL NEED

250 ml (8½ fl oz/1 cup) water

1 teaspoon sage leaves (3–4 leaves)

GET STARTED

Bring the water to the boil in a small saucepan. Put the
sage leaves in a cup and pour the water over them.

Leave to infuse for 10 minutes, then strain and drink.

This tea can also be used for gargling — do this twice
a day.

WHY WE BELIEVE IT WORKS

The word sage can be traced back to the Latin word
salvare, which means 'healing'. The essential oils
contained in sage leaves are anti-inflammatory,
fungicidal, virus-inhibiting and antibacterial.

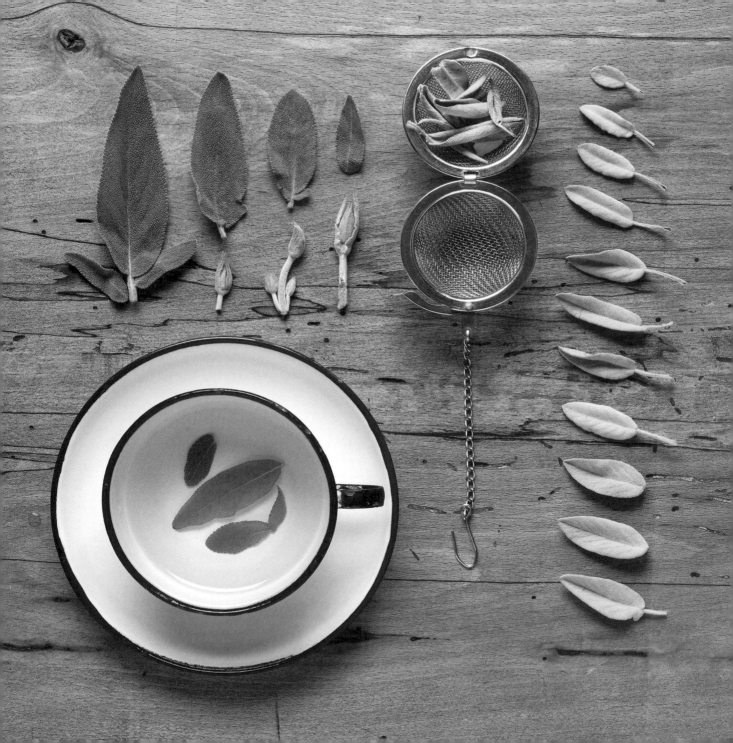

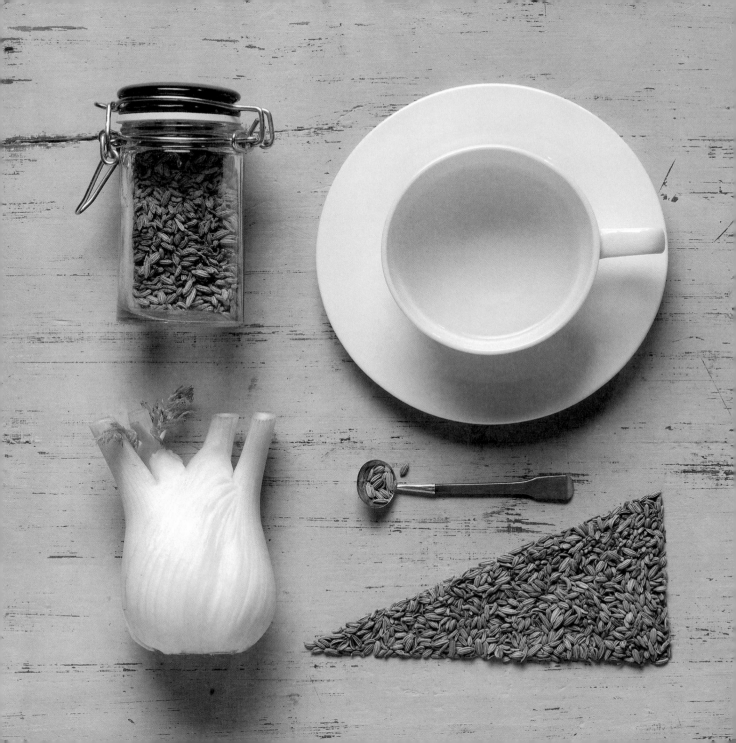

FENNEL TEA

Helps with inflammation in the mouth and throat

THINGS YOU'LL NEED

1 teaspoon fennel seeds, or ¼ fennel bulb, diced

250 ml (8½ fl oz/1 cup) water

This tea is very soothing for infections of the mouth or throat. I drink several cups of it daily when I'm feeling ill. An additional effect is that it helps to treat flatulence. You can use fennel seeds or a fresh fennel bulb for the infusion, but the healing properties are strongest in the seeds.

– KARIN

GET STARTED

Put the fennel seeds in a cup. Bring the water to the boil and pour over the seeds, leave to infuse for 10 minutes. Strain into a cup and drink.

WHY WE BELIEVE IT WORKS

Fennel is high in vitamin C and contains antibacterial essences, which are anti-inflammatory. It loosens phlegm and has antispasmodic and antiseptic properties. Fennel also has a calming effect on the stomach and gut. In Austria, fennel tea is very popular and is given to babies with abdominal bloating and colic.

WHITE RADISH SOUP

Feed a cold, starve a fever

THINGS YOU'LL NEED

4–5 spring onions (scallions), finely
sliced

15 g (½ oz) fresh ginger, finely sliced

1 white radish, finely sliced

1 litre (34 fl oz/4 cups) water

This soup should help you to sweat away all symptoms of your cold in no time. Isn't it great when the cure is also dinner?

– NICI

GET STARTED

Place the spring onions, ginger and radish in a saucepan. Add the water and bring to the boil.

Reduce the heat slightly and simmer for 10 minutes or until the water has reduced to one-third of the original amount.

Grab a spoon and enjoy this delicious, healing soup for lunch or dinner or whenever you feel like it.

WHY WE BELIEVE IT WORKS

Spring onions act as an antiseptic and are also anti-inflammatory.

Ginger has antibiotic properties and stimulates the immune system.

White radish encourages sweating, is antibacterial and fungicidal and loosens phlegm.

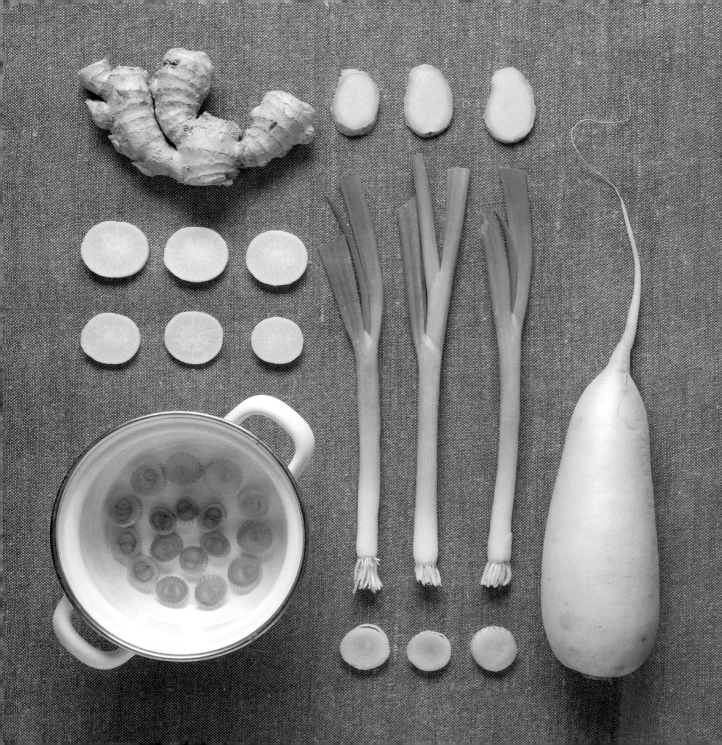

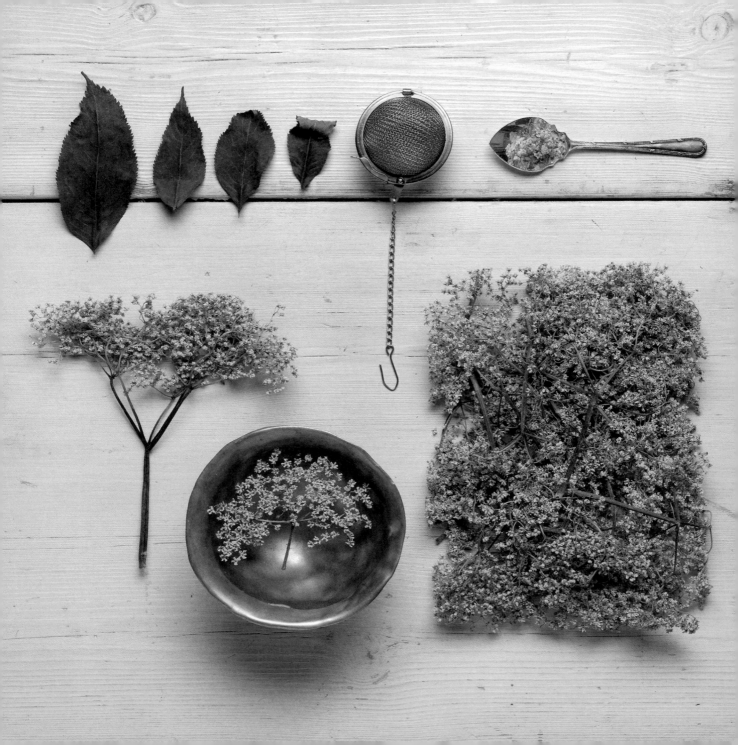

ELDERFLOWER INFUSION

We use this for coughs and sinusitis

The elderberry bush only flowers for a few weeks each year between May and July. You can easily miss this if you don't live near one, like my dad, who collected the flowers in the picture. However, they can be sourced online or in health food shops. The fragrance is truly wonderful. Elderflower essences have been valued since ancient Greece. According to folklore, the elderberry bush wards off evil spirits, and cutting the bush down leads to bad luck.

– KARIN

THINGS YOU'LL NEED

1 tablespoon elderflowers

250 ml (8½ fl oz/1 cup) water

GET STARTED

Put the elderflowers in a cup and pour boiling water over them.

Leave to infuse for 10 minutes, then strain into a cup and drink straight away.

To prevent a cold, drink one cup of this tea up to three times daily as soon as you notice any symptoms. This will boost your metabolism and immune system.

WHY WE BELIEVE IT WORKS

An infusion of elderflowers encourages the body to sweat and lowers fever. It also dissolves mucus and eases colds, irritable coughs and bronchial catarrh. Elderflowers also have anti-inflammatory properties.

POTATO WRAP

I use this for coughs
and bronchitis

THINGS YOU'LL NEED

3 medium potatoes, unpeeled

1 tea towel (dish cloth)

With a stubborn cough or bronchitis, it's all about
getting warm and toasty. Nothing will deliver the heat
you need better than everyone's favourite comfort food:
the potato.

– NICI

GET STARTED

Boil the potatoes and mash them. Leave to cool for
2–3 minutes.

Now for the tricky part: do not eat! Instead, fold the
tea towel lengthways into a long strip. Unfold one layer
and arrange the mashed potatos along the length of the
towel.

Fold the towel over the mashed potatoes and tuck in the
sides so the potato stays inside.

Either wrap this around your neck and secure with a
scarf or lie down and place the wrap on the bare skin of
your chest.

Important: make sure the wrap is not too hot, to avoid
burning yourself.

WHY WE BELIEVE IT WORKS

Potato wraps help loosen phlegm and are pain-relieving
and warming.

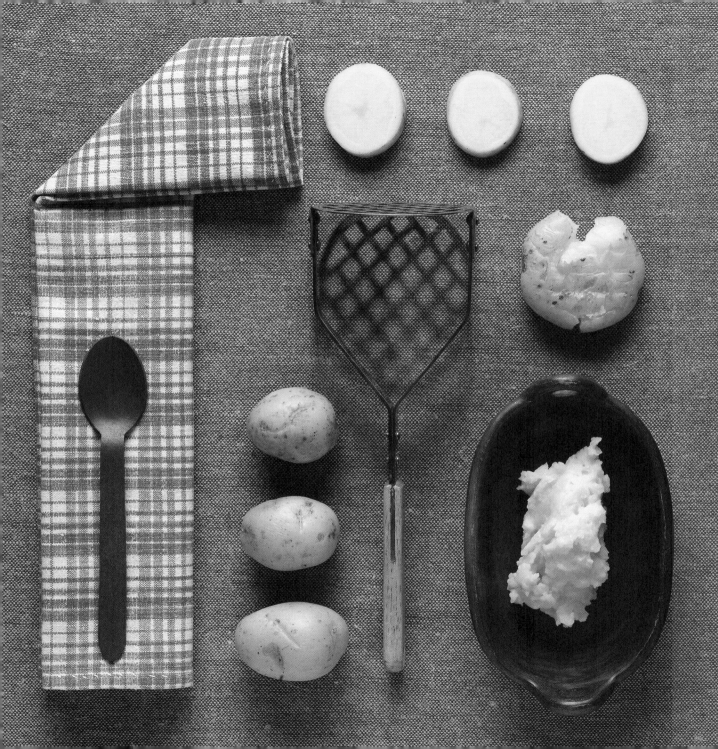

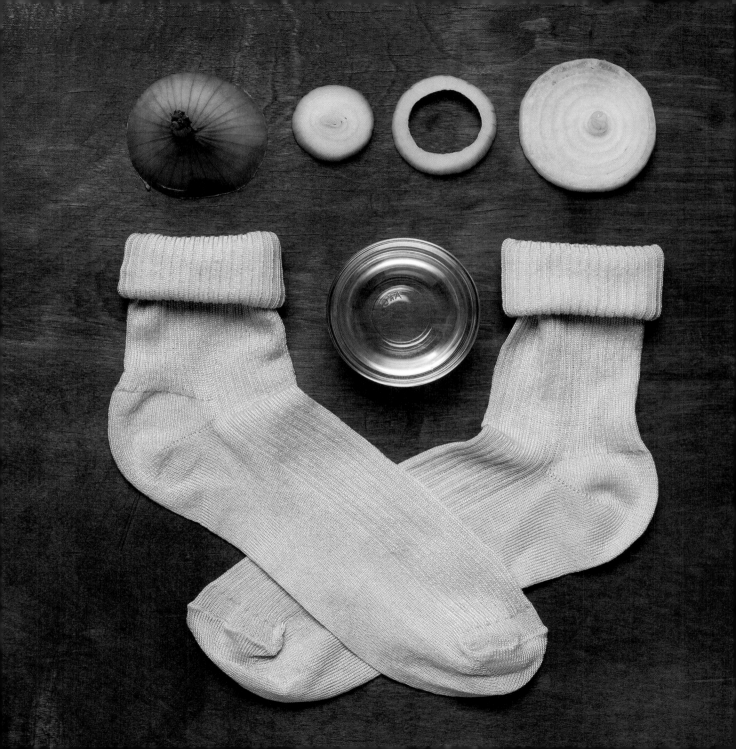

ONION SOCKS

Fun remedy for fevers and colds

THINGS YOU'LL NEED

1 onion, sliced

cotton wool

gauze bandages

safety pins

lovely warm, wool socks

hot water bottle (optional)

... a helping hand!

Sometimes, in the battle against fever and colds no measure is too peculiar – or, in this case, too much fun!

– NICI

GET STARTED

Heat some water in a pan until boiling. Place the onion slices in a sieve and warm them by carefully holding the sieve over the steaming water.

Now, for this part you might need a helping hand: place the warmed onion slices on the soles of your feet and cover with a thin layer of cotton wool.

Secure in place with gauze bandages and a small safety pin. That's the tricky bit done! Put on the woolly socks and walk around, so the essential oils are absorbed through your skin.

If the fever isn't too high, you could even risk a little dance move – as long as you lie down right after! To keep the onions warm, put a hot water bottle by your feet.

WHY WE BELIEVE IT WORKS

Once absorbed through the skin, the essential oils have an anti-inflammatory effect. Onions have antibacterial as well as antiseptic properties, they also are a great immune booster.

THYME, PEPPERMINT & RIBWORT PLANTAIN INFUSION

Try this for bronchitis

I have this mixture prepared and ready to use whenever I feel bronchitis coming on. Ribwort plantain leaf is an unfamiliar plant to most people. Although it does grow outside my mum's kitchen, we had to order it online for this image. However, once you know what it looks like you'll see it growing everywhere!

– KARIN

THINGS YOU'LL NEED

1 teaspoon thyme leaves

3 teaspoons peppermint leaves
(9–12 leaves)

2 teaspoons ribwort plantain
leaves (6–8 leaves)

saucepan

250 ml (8½ fl oz/1 cup) water

honey, to taste (optional)

GET STARTED

Mix the thyme, peppermint and ribwort plantain leaves. Put 1 teaspoon of this herb mix in a saucepan.

Boil the water and pour over the herbs. Leave to infuse for 10–15 minutes, then strain into a clean glass. Just before drinking, sweeten with honey if desired.

WHY WE BELIEVE IT WORKS

Thyme helps to loosen phlegm. Peppermint is soothing, antispasmodic and pain-relieving. Ribwort plantain leaves have antibiotic properties.

Honey helps to loosen phlegm, is antibacterial and nutritious.

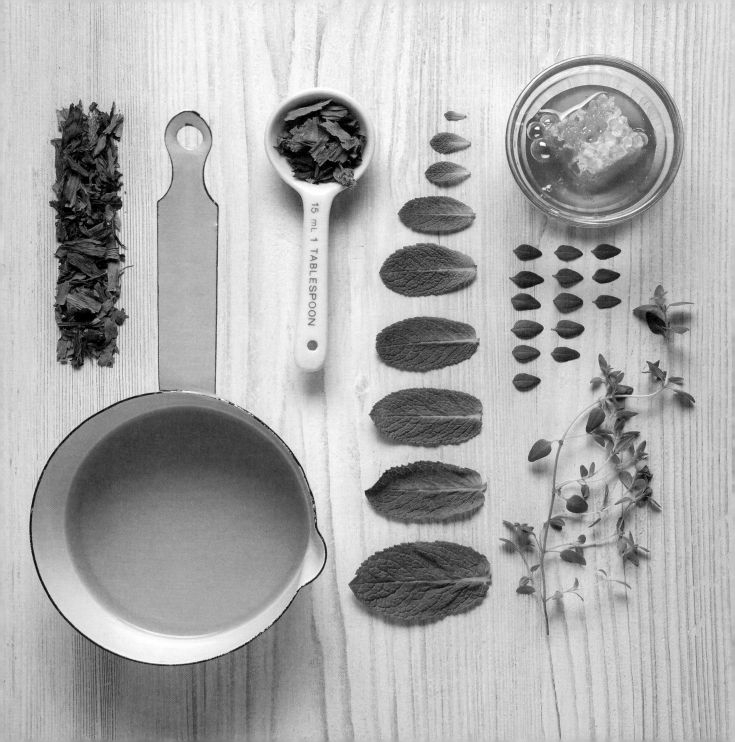

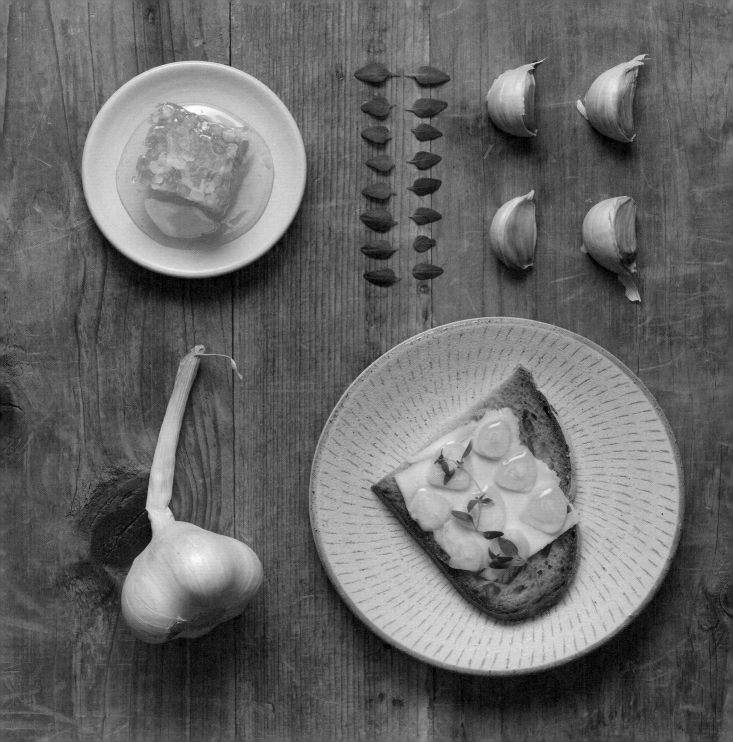

GARLIC BREAD WITH HONEY & THYME

Mum's answer for colds

THINGS YOU'LL NEED

butter

bread

2-3 cloves garlic, peeled and
finely sliced

honey

thyme leaves

This recipe is an effective and easily prepared cure for colds. If your mum never made this for you, don't be put off by the unusual mix of ingredients. Eating raw garlic might make you smelly, but this yummy recipe means that you can benefit from all its goodness while enjoying something really tasty. You'll find that smelling of garlic for one day is a small price to pay. You could use dried thyme if you can't get hold of fresh, but thyme really is something everyone should have in their window box.

– KARIN

GET STARTED

Spread some butter on a slice of bread, add the garlic, dribble some honey over the top and sprinkle with thyme leaves.

WHY WE BELIEVE IT WORKS

Three powerful natural drugs on one slice of bread will give a boost to even the weakest immune system.

Garlic is a natural antibiotic and strengthens the immune system. It has been highly regarded for centuries and it was even used as a burial object for the pharaohs in ancient Egypt.

Honey is very nutritious and is a remedy that dates back to the ancient Greeks. Honey was and still is used as a wound-healing ointment. Honey strengthens the immune system, prevents bacterial growth and reduces fever. It is antimicrobial, and full of antioxidants.

Thyme is antibacterial, fungicidal and antiviral. It strengthens the immune system, supports the digestive system and boosts blood circulation.

FERN LINIMENT

We treat pain, rheumatism
and headaches with this

THINGS YOU'LL NEED

handful of wood fern roots

1 preserving jar

1 litre (34 fl oz/4 cups) rubbing alcohol

1 dark glass bottle

According to legend, the mysterious wood fern plant was
thought to be the secret to invisibility. So here's how
to become invisible in a few simple steps. But wait —
first I'll tell you how to get rid of aches and pains.

– NICI

GET STARTED

First, wash and clean any earth off the fern roots,
then cut them into small pieces.

Fill the jar with the rubbing alcohol and add the fern
root. Seal the jar and leave in a cool, dark place.
After 4 weeks, strain the liquid into a dark glass
bottle — the dark glass keeps the light out, allowing
the liniment to stay potent for longer.

Gently rub a little of the liniment onto areas where you
feel back pain, rheumatism, arthritis or headaches to
make them ... disappear.

WHY WE BELIEVE IT WORKS

Ferns have been widely used since medieval times.
They contain tannins which are antispasmodic and
anti-inflammatory.

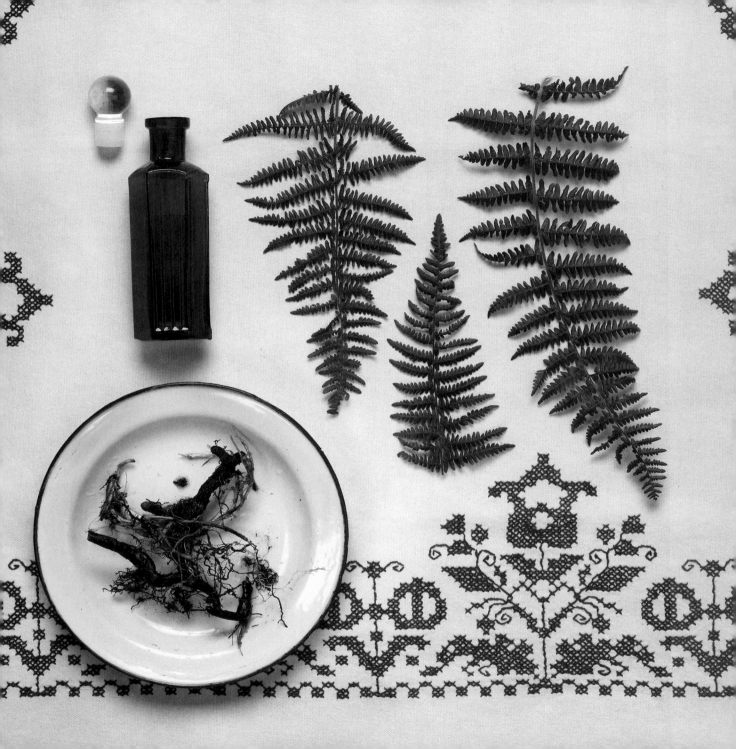

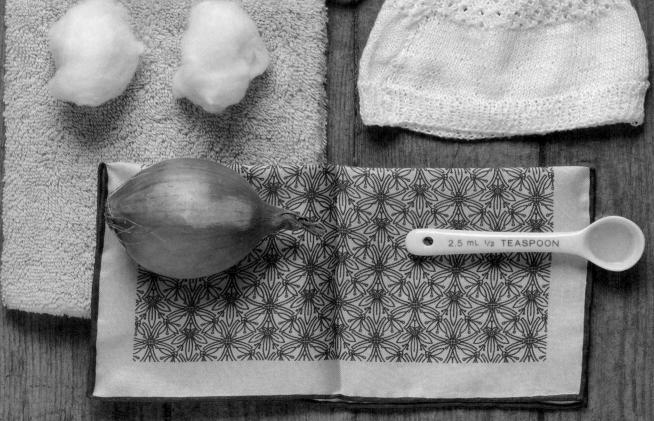

ONION
HAT

For ear infections

THINGS YOU'LL NEED

1 onion

cotton handkerchief

face flannel

woolly hat

St John's wort oil

cotton wool

If your ear hurts, you might be wearing a woolly hat already. All that's missing now is some onion to really make the pain go away. Sounds peculiar? Maybe – but this is one of our secret weapons, so give it a try!

– NICI

GET STARTED

Finely slice or dice the onion. Place the onion pieces on the handkerchief and fold into a firm little parcel.

Now dip a face flannel into some hot water and squeeze out any excess water. Place the onion parcel against your ear, cover with the flannel and secure with a woolly hat. Sit down and relax for 20 minutes. You'll probably feel a bit silly, but also quite smug, knowing this will do the trick.

Remove the compress and put 2 drops of St John's wort oil in your ear. Finish the treatment by carefully placing a small ball of cotton wool in your ear.

Repeat the ritual for 2–3 days on both ears. Even if only one ear hurts this must, for some reason, be done on both sides. Always!

WHY WE BELIEVE IT WORKS

Chopped onions release antibacterial as well as disinfecting substances and reduce inflammation.
St John's wort oil is anti-inflammatory, antibacterial, soothing and pain-relieving.

CONKER BATHING ESSENCE

For rheumatism and gout; encourages blood circulation

On some playgrounds of the world it's all about conkers and string, but it is conkers and toothpicks in Austria... Conkers are used as the heads and bodies, with toothpicks for necks and legs – there are no limits to your extensive conkers zoo you always dreamed of! But calm yourself, the only 'conkimal' you'll need for this recipe is a conker-duck to replace your loyal rubber bath companion.

– NICI

THINGS YOU'LL NEED (FOR A FULL BATH)

half a bucket of ripe conkers (horse chestnuts), around 900 g (2 lb)

enough water to cover the conkers

GET STARTED

First, remove the spiky shell from the conkers. (Try to resist threading string through those shiny beauties for a conker contest!)

Cut the conkers into small pieces and soak them in a large saucepan of water overnight, until soft. The next day, bring the conkers and water to the boil. Remove from the heat and allow to infuse for 10 minutes. Strain the liquid into a clean bowl.

Add the strained liquid to your bath. Give it a little stir – this should produce foam because of the saponins.

My grandad took this relaxing bath once a week during chestnut season.

WHY WE BELIEVE IT WORKS

Conkers (also known as horse chestnuts) are antibacterial, anti-inflammatory, astringent and antispasmodic. They also cleanse the blood.

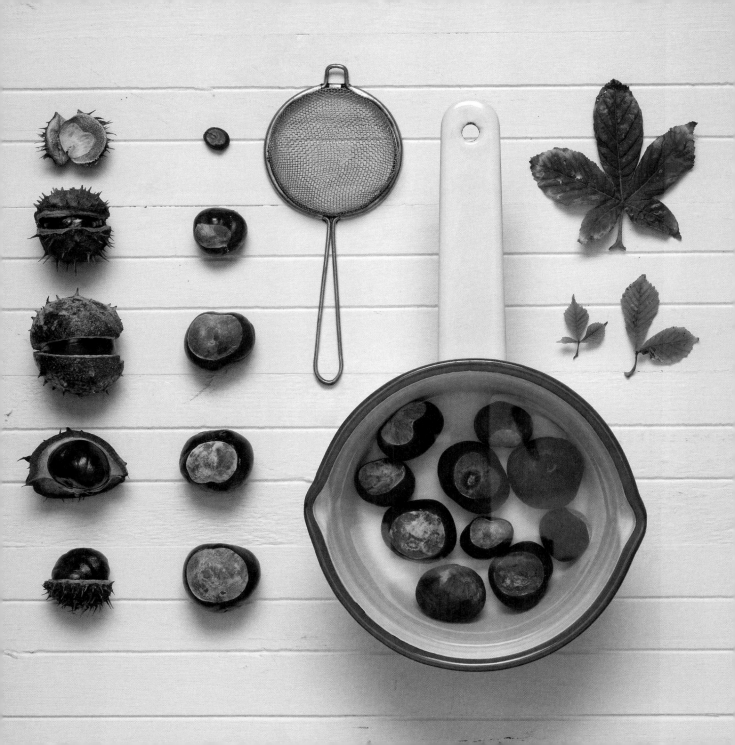

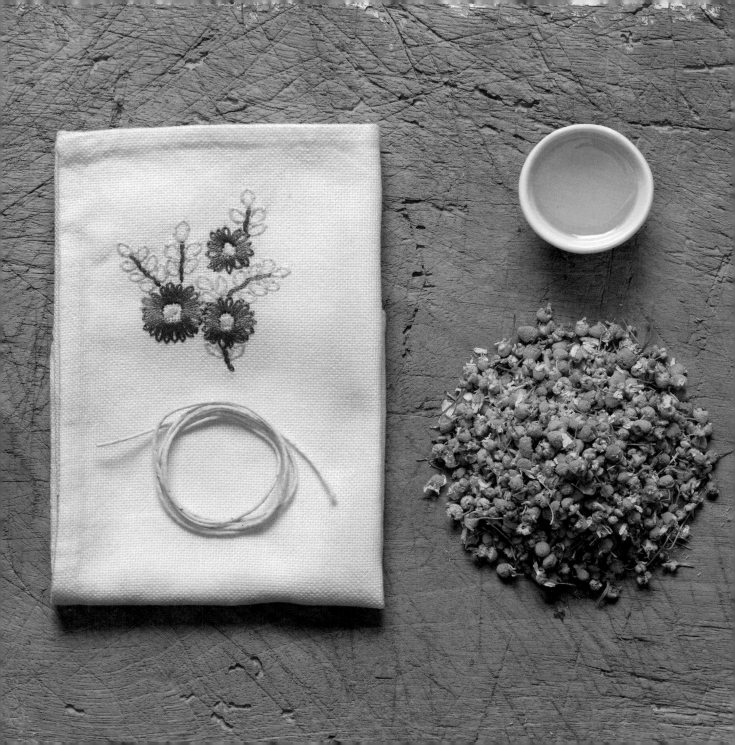

CHAMOMILE PARCEL

Our secret to unblocking sinuses

THINGS YOU'LL NEED

1 hot water bottle

chamomile flowers

square linen cloth

string

towel

marigold oil or St John's wort oil

This traditional remedy is a bit like making a layer cake (with you as the cake base). It will both sooth and unblock inflamed sinuses. All you need to do is layer up. The best time for this is at night, just before going to bed.

– NICI

GET STARTED

Prepare your hot water bottle.

Put a handful of chamomile flowers in the centre of the linen cloth and fold into a little sachet, then secure it with the string. Dip the sachet into some hot water – a bit like dunking a very large tea bag.

Lie down, make sure you are comfortable, and start layering: for the first layer, place the chamomile sachet over your sinuses. For the second layer, place the towel on top, so the heat and steam can work on your sinuses. For the third layer, place the hot water bottle on top of the towel to keep all the layers warm and steamy. Relax. Breathe. Have a little rest.

After 15 minutes, remove all the layers and rub the sinus area gently with either marigold oil or St John's wort oil. Now go straight to bed.

WHY WE BELIEVE IT WORKS

Chamomile is anti-inflammatory and antispasmodic. It also has mild antibacterial qualities.

The saponins in marigold oil reduce swelling. It also contains flavonoids, which are anti-inflammatory, and carotenoids (yellow and orange pigments) which promote the formation of new tissue.

St John's wort oil is anti-inflammatory and famous for its wound-healing properties.

PRUNE INFUSION

This often helps constipation

THINGS YOU'LL NEED

handful of prunes

750 ml (25 fl oz/3 cups) water

So ... nothing's happening for an unusually long period of time? Fear not. Prunes are a natural way to get things going!

– NICI

GET STARTED

Soak the prunes and in the water overnight. The next morning, or after around 12 hours, strain the juice into a cup and sip it slowly. The soft prunes can be cut into small pieces and added to the juice for dietary fibre, which also helps with digestion.

WHY WE BELIEVE IT WORKS

As well as being a natural laxative and full of vitamins, prunes are high in antioxidants and contain fluoride, iron and potassium. Potassium regulates blood pressure and keeps blood sugar stable.

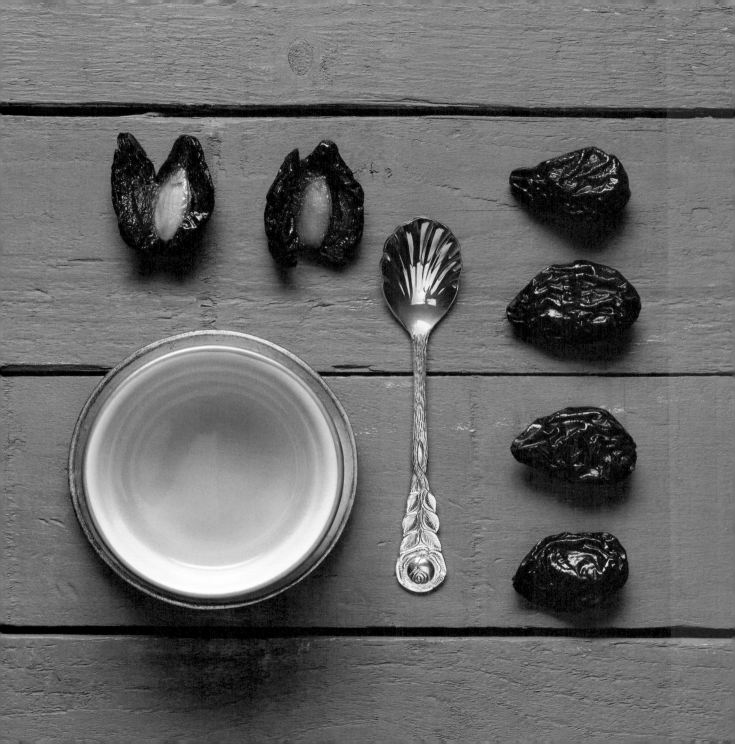

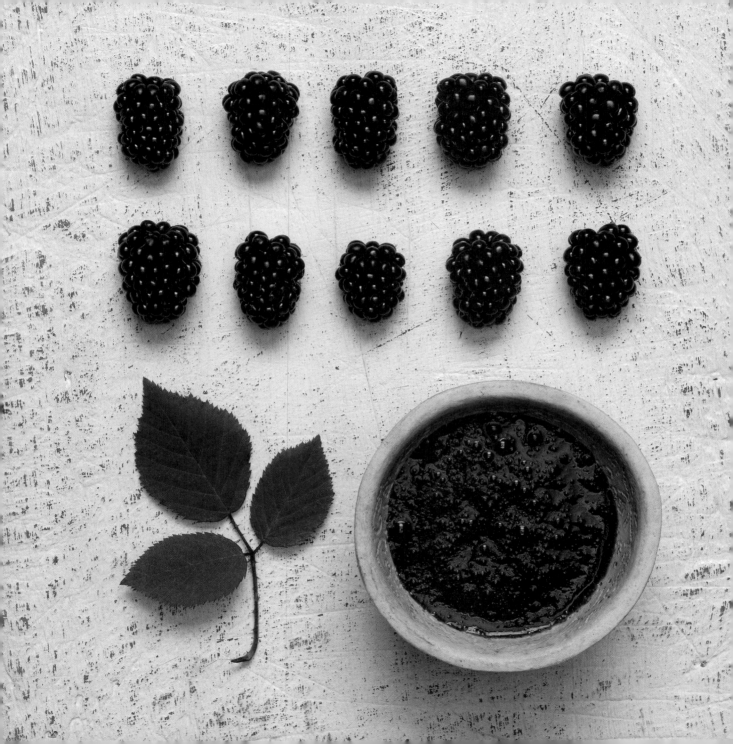

BLACKBERRY JUICE

Try this at the first signs
of a sore throat

This is so delicious you'll want to make it even when
you are not suffering from a sore throat. Be sure
to warm the juice slightly before sipping if the
blackberries have been sitting in the fridge — it should
only be consumed at room temperature. Before swallowing,
sip and chew slowly or gargle, so that the juice stays
in the mouth long enough for the saliva (which has
antibacterial properties) to work its magic.

– KARIN

THINGS YOU'LL NEED

150g (5oz/1 cup) blackberries

GET STARTED

Put the blackberries in a strainer and squash them
carefully with the back of a spoon over a clean glass to
extract the juice. Don't discard the squashed berries
left behind in the strainer — they're delicious, too!

We found that a tea strainer was much quicker to use than
a sieve, and there was hardly any washing up. This recipe
will give you around 125 ml (4 fl oz/½ cup) juice.

WHY WE BELIEVE IT WORKS

Blackberries are astringent, cleanse the blood and
are high in Vitamin C, which make them ideal for
treating inflammation of the mucous membranes in the
mouth and throat.

LIME BLOSSOM INFUSION

We use this for fever and irritating coughs

Lime trees, also known as linden, are not to be confused with the trees that bear lime fruit. They grow to a very old age and were usually planted close to populated areas. Lime trees were thought to be holy, and during the Middle Ages judicial hearings were held under them.

I pick the flowers and upper leaves (the long, thin leaf attached to the flower) from lime trees that grow near my home up to five days after they first blossom. The flowers appear in July and have a lovely, subtle smell. Drink this fragrant tea whenever you have a chesty cough.

– KARIN

THINGS YOU'LL NEED

1 teaspoon lime blossoms

250 ml (8½ fl oz/1 cup) water

GET STARTED

Put the blossoms in a saucepan and pour boiling water over them.

Leave to infuse for 10 minutes, then strain into a cup and drink immediately. The taste is mildly sweet.

WHY WE BELIEVE IT WORKS

Lime blossom contains essential oils, flavonoids, saponins and mucilages.

A lime blossom infusion is anti-inflammatory, antispasmodic, pain-relieving and eases sore throats. It also has a calming effect, which is useful in treating an upset stomach, cramps and mild migraines.

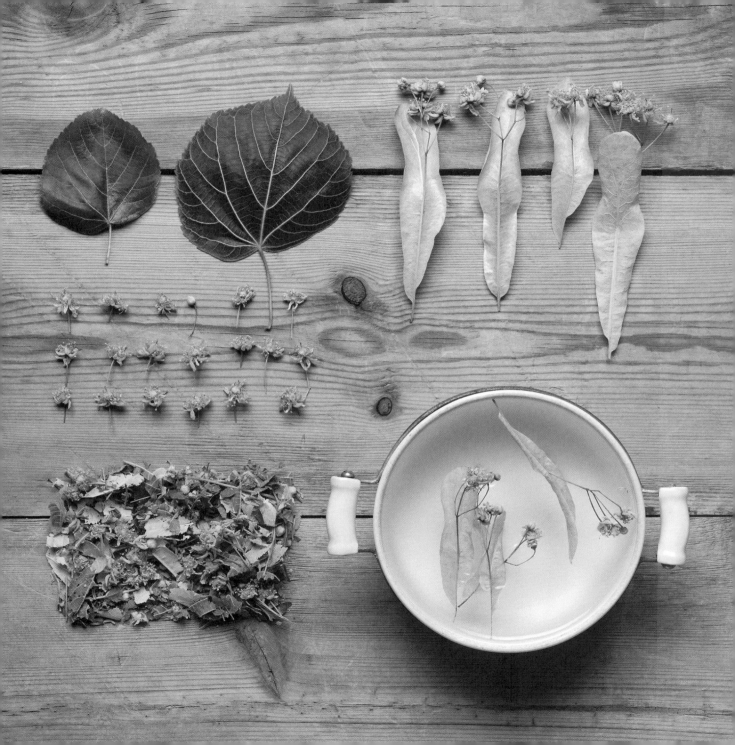

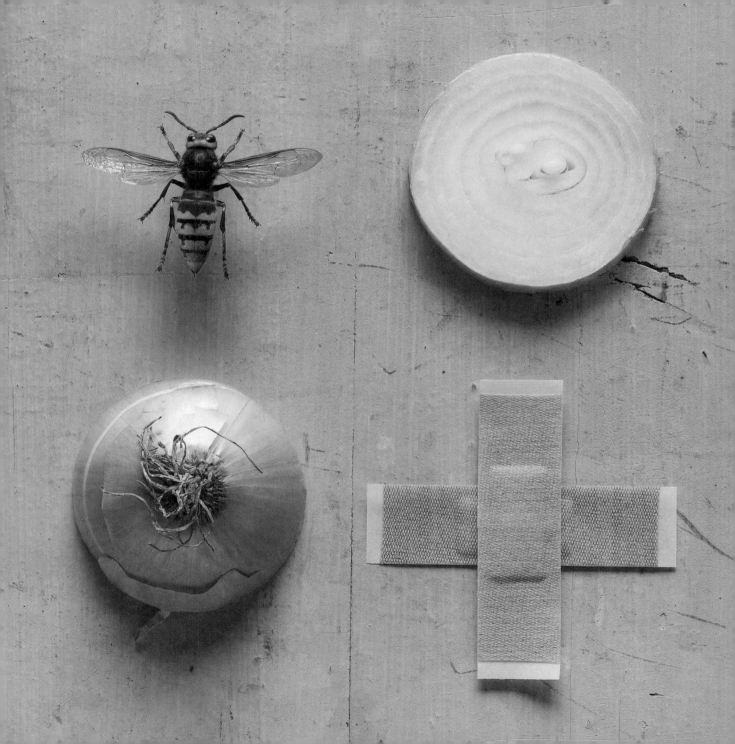

ONION REMEDY

Traditional remedy for
a bee or wasp sting

I haven't been stung by a bee for a long time. As a child though, I remember running through the grass in bare feet and stepping on and getting stung by a bee or wasp at least every other summer. Onions are an inexpensive ingredient for every home medicine chest and are a real panacea.

– KARIN

THINGS YOU'LL NEED

tweezers

1 onion, halved

GET STARTED

Remove the bee's stinger with tweezers and immediately rub the freshly cut side of the onion-half over the stung area.

WHY WE BELIEVE IT WORKS

Onions contain flavonoids, some of which are known to reduce inflammation. Onions are also anti-inflammatory and antibacterial and have disinfecting properties.

CARAWAY, FENNEL & ANISEED INFUSION

Helps flatulence

Caraway is probably Europe's oldest medicinal plant and spice and has been in use for thousands of years. Enjoy a cup of this infusion whenever your digestive tract is in trouble.

– KARIN

THINGS YOU'LL NEED

2 tablespoons caraway seeds

2 tablespoons fennel seeds

2 tablespoons, aniseeds
or Chinese star anise

250ml (8½ fl oz/1 cup) water

GET STARTED

Mix the crushed seeds together and put 2 teaspoons of this seed mixture in a cup. Bring the water to the boil and pour into a cup. Leave to infuse for 10 minutes, then strain and drink unsweetened.

Store the remaining seed mixture in a cool, dark, dry place until you need it again.

WHY WE BELIEVE IT WORKS

The essential oils found in caraway seeds are known to have antioxidant, digestive and carminative (anti-flatulence) properties.

Aniseed and star anise both contain an essential oil called anethole which has strong antimicrobial qualities. It can also improve digestion and ease flatulence.

Fennel seeds have similar properties to aniseed and can also help to treat flatulence. Fennel seeds are antibacterial, antispasmodic and anti-inflamatory.

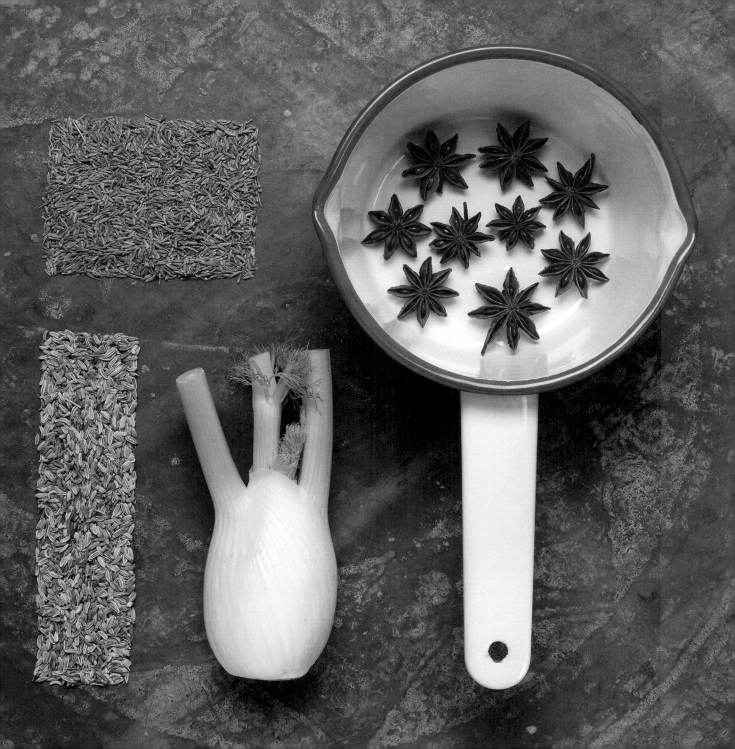

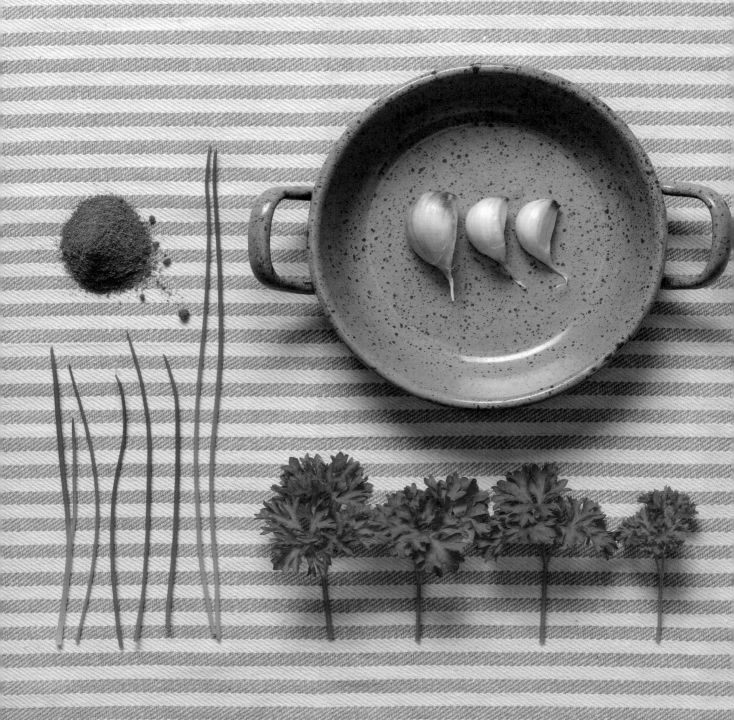

GARLIC, CAYENNE PEPPER, PARSLEY & CHIVE INFUSION

Combats fatigue

This curious remedy is a tea with soup ingredients. One ingredient in this recipe, which can't be found growing naturally in our native Austria, is cayenne pepper. Still, it has sneaked its way into this book!

– KARIN

THINGS YOU'LL NEED

250 ml (8½ fl oz/1 cup) water

2 garlic cloves, peeled

3 sprigs of fresh parsley

3 fresh chives

1 pinch of cayenne pepper

GET STARTED

Place a small pan on the stove with the water. Bring the water to the boil, remove from the heat and add the garlic. Allow to infuse for 10 minutes.

Finely chop the parsley and chives and add to the infusion. Then finish off with the cayenne pepper. Strain into a cup or small bowl and drink as hot as you can, without burning your tongue.

WHY WE BELIEVE IT WORKS

The antibacterial and disinfectant properties of garlic combined with the stimulating and antispasmodic properties of parsley work wonders.

Chives are high in Vitamin C, are blood-cleansing and loosen phlegm.

Cayenne pepper stimulates circulation and is cleansing and detoxifying. It also helps to fight off infection and inflammation.

ROSE & VINEGAR SOLUTION

For fatigue and faintness

THINGS YOU'LL NEED

petals from 2-3 roses

750 ml-1 litre (25-34 fl oz) wide-necked jar

500 ml (17fl oz/2 cups) vinegar

1 glass bottle

Rub this lovely mixture over your whole body after a shower or whenever you're feeling tired and exhausted.

Pick the roses just before they start to unfold. This is when the level of essential oils in rose petals is at its highest. Only use roses that haven't been sprayed with pesticides.

– KARIN

GET STARTED

Place the petals in the jar, add the undiluted vinegar, and cover with the lid.

Store in a cool, dry place for 14 days, out of sunlight, and shake the jar once a day.

Strain the liquid into a sterilized glass bottle. Its lovely, bright colours will make this a very happy experience!

WHY WE BELIEVE IT WORKS

The essential oils in rose petals help to support the nervous system and are anti-inflammatory, astringent and blood cleansing.

Vinegar is disinfecting and antibacterial, and helps wounds to heal. It stimulates circulation, is anti-inflammatory and boosts the metabolism.

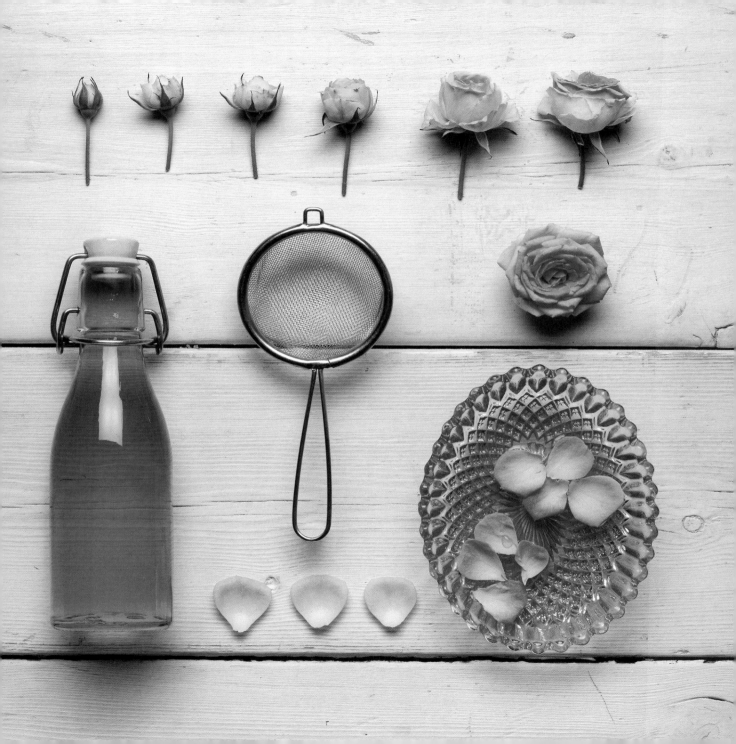

KEY INGREDIENTS

A little collection of the ingrediences in this book and why we and our ancestors believe they work. Some scientists agree, some don't - so best to test for yourself after talking to your doctor.

Aniseeds: contain an essential oil called anethole which has strong antimicrobial qualities. Aniseeds can improve digestion and ease flatulence. They are antibacterial and anticonvulsant while their cleansing properties have a beneficial effect on many chronic illnesses.

Apple cider vinegar: stimulates blood flow, boosts the immune system and helps waste products to break down faster. It supports natural bodily functions and aids metabolism and the absorption of important nutrients from food. It improves digestion and blood circulation. It is anti-inflammatory, antibacterial, disinfecting, supports wound healing, prevents the spread of putrefactive bacteria in the gut, improves kidney performance and tightens tissue and skin.

Apples: high in nutritional value. Apples contain vitamins A, B1, B2, B6, E, C and folic acid, and trace elements and minerals such as potassium. The fruit acids in apples inhibit harmful enzymes and putrefactive bacteria in the gut as well as aid digestion.

Beeswax: antibiotic, anti-inflammatory, antiseptic and rich in vitamin A which boosts skin cell production.

Blackberries: are astringent, cleanse the blood and are high in vitamin C, which makes them ideal for treating inflammation of the mucous membranes in the mouth and throat.

Blueberries: dried berries and leaves contain tannins, which have an astringent effect and prevent essential nutrients from getting lost in your gut when you suffer from diarrhoea.

Buttermilk: has anti-inflammatory properties, and is healing and cooling on the skin.

Caraway seeds: the essential oils have antioxidant, digestive and carminative (antiflatulence) properties.

Cayenne pepper: stimulates circulation, is cleansing and detoxifying.

Chamomile: disinfects and has anti-inflammatory, antibacterial and antispasmodic properties. It also acts as a sedative and relieves anxiety and insomnia.

Chives: high in vitamin C, chives are also blood cleansing and loosen phlegm.

Conkers (horsechestnuts): antibacterial, anti-inflammatory, blood cleansing, astringent and antispasmodic.

Curd cheese: anti-inflammatory and soothing to the digestion. It contains minerals and vitamins, will boost the metabolism, soothes pain and is cooling to the skin. When curd comes in contact with skin, a lactic acid process is triggered, which opens the pores and stimulates blood flow. The inflammation is absorbed by the curd. When the curd warms up due to your body heat, it also helps to dissolve phlegm.

Dandelions: are detoxifying and stimulate the metabolism.

Elderflower: encourages the body to sweat and is believed to lower fever. It dissolves phlegm and eases colds, irritable coughs and bronchial catarrh. It also has anti-inflammatory properties.

Fennel and fennel seeds: high in vitamin C, with antibacterial, anti-inflammatory, antispasmodic and antiseptic properties. Fennel helps to loosen phlegm and has a calming effect on the stomach and gut. Good for treating flatulence.

Garlic: A superfood. A natural antibiotic, with anitoxidant, antifungal, antiviral, immune-boosting and disinfectant properties. Contains vitamin C, Manganese, B6 and is believed to lower cholesterol and blood-pressure. Some studies have shown that garlic may offer some protection against cancer.

Ginger: stimulates the immune system, lowers cholesterol and has antibiotic and anti-inflammatory properties.

Honey: a mild and natural laxative. Honey strengthens the immune system, prevents bacterial growth and reduces fever. Honey is wound healing. It is antispasmodic and anticonvulsant, and acts as an expectorant, dissolving mucus. Honey is nutritious and invigorating but very sensitive to heat. Always use the most natural honey you can find: organic, raw honey is the best.

Horseradish: lowers fever and is a traditional remedy for unblocking airways. It acts as an antibiotic and has antiviral properties. Horseradish contains vitamins C and B1, and flavonoids. It dissolves mucus, is antimicrobial and stimulates blood flow.

Larch sap: helps skin to heal, prevents infection, and provides relief for rheumatism, blisters, insect bites and corns.

Lavender: the essential oil is relaxing and soothing. Lavender also has anti-inflammatory and antiseptic properties that help heal wounds.

Lemons: antibacterial, antiviral, body-cleansing, infection-fighting, rich in vitamin C and flavonoids.

Lime blossom: anti-inflammatory, antispasmodic and pain-relieving. Lime blossom has a calming effect, which is useful in treating digestive tract troubles, cramps and mild migraines. The essential oil contains flavonoids and saponins. The mucilages, or secretions, ease coughs.

Linseeds: aid digestion, protect the lining of the intestines and are rich in dietary fibre. They are also high in minerals and vitamins.

Marigold oil: contains saponins which reduces swelling, flavonoids, which are anti-inflammatory and carotenoids which promote the formation of new tissue.

Mustard seeds: pain-relieving and anticonvulsant. Mustard seeds can be used to treat inflammation, rheumatism and headaches.

Nettles: these act as a tonic, are anti-allergenic, antispasmodic, blood-cleansing, blood-building, and high in vitamin C and iron. They also have antihistamine properties and have been used in the treatment of diabetes and eczema. Nettles can be helpful in relieving the pain of arthritis.

Olive oil: contains antioxidants and vitamin E.

Onions: have antibacterial, anti-inflammatory and disinfecting properties. They contain antioxidants and flavonoids and help to thin the blood, detoxify the body and lower cholesterol. They have been shown to be beneficial for sufferers of diabetes and arthritis.

Parsley: a natural stimulant, with antispasmodic and anti-inflammatory properties. It also contains flavonoids, vitamin C and zinc.

Pepper: freshly ground pepper stimulates the circulation and digestive system. Pepper is antibacterial and works as a decongestant.

Peppermint: soothing, antispasmodic, antimicrobial and pain-relieving. Peppermint also helps ease congested airways.

Peony flowers: antispasmodic and anti-inflammatory.

Potatoes: pain-relieving, warming and helpful in dissolving mucus.

Prunes: laxative, full of vitamins and antioxidants. Prunes contain fluoride, iron and potassium, which regulates blood pressure and stabilizes blood sugar.

Quince: rich in vitamin C, iodine and zinc as well as mucilages.

Radishes (white and black mooli or daikon radish): antibacterial, fungicidal, encourage sweating and help to dissolve mucus. Black mooli contains healing minerals and vitamins which have antimicrobial and antiviral properties and strengthen the immune system.

Ribwort plantain: the leaves have antibiotic properties and are astringent, wound-healing and blood-purifying.

Roses: anti-inflammatory, astringent and blood cleansing.

Rosemary: aids digestion, is appetising and has carminative properties. It is cardiotonic (good for the heart), cleanses the blood, and has antibacterial and antispasmodic properties.

Sage: its essential oil is anti-inflammatory, antibacterial, fungicidal and virus-inhibiting.

St John's wort oil: anti-inflammatory and antibacterial, with soothing, pain-relieving, wound-healing properties.

Sea salt: the main constituents of sea salt are magnesium, potassium, calcium, iodine, bromine and iron. Salt helps loosens phlegm, strengthens your immune system, and acts as a disinfectant.

Spring onions: are antiseptic and anti-inflammatory.

Spruce needles: have an invigorating and antispasmodic effect and stimulate the blood flow. Their essential oils clear and disinfect the lungs and airways.

Star anise (Chinese): contain an essential oil called anethole which has strong antimicrobial qualities. Star anise has antibacterial, antioxidant and antifungal benefits. It can also improve digestion and ease flatulence.

Thyme: antibacterial, disinfecting, anti-inflammatory, fungicidal and anti-viral. It strengthens our immune system, supports the digestive system, boosts blood circulation and helps to loosen phlegm.

Valerian: calming, relaxing and soporific.

Wood fern: the essential oils are antispasmodic and anti-inflammatory. Can be used to treat gout and alleviate rheumatism. *Only use externally.*

GLOSSARY

Anti-bacterial: destructive to or inhibiting the growth of bacteria.

Anti-microbial: destructive to or inhibiting the growth of microorganisms.

Anti-oxidants: Substances that have the potential to prevent oxidative damage to cell membranes, DNA and other celular macromolecules, when free radical activity outweighs the cell's own antioxidant defense mechanisms.

Antiseptic: inhibits growth or reproduction of micro-organisms including bacteria, funghi and viruses.

Anti-spasmodic: loosens muscle spasms.

Anti-viral: supressing the virus' ability to multiply and reproduce.

Astringent: causing contraction of soft tissue.

Cardiotonic: having a beneficial effect on the heart.

Carminative: combatting flatulence.

Clavus: hard thickening of the skin.

Flavonoids: is a group of phytonutrients that are anti-allergenic, anti-inflammatory, anti-oxidant, anti-microbial and have anti-diarrheal properties.

Fungicidal: destructive to or inhibiting the growth of fungi.

Mucilages: plant secretions capable of easing cough.

Mucous dissolving: loosens phlegm.

Mucous membranes: lubricating membranes inside the mouth, for example.

Putrefactive: rotting.

Soporific: causes drowsiness.

Saponins: natural compounds, found in many plants, with detergent and emulsifying properties.

Topfen: curd cheese or quark.

AILMENT INDEX

Page references in *italics* are recipe entries

INDEX

Page references in *italics* are recipe entries

THANK YOUS
DANKESCHÖNS

Our special thanks go to Regina, who provided valuable advice, many of the recipes, and perfectly dried herbs in this book. To Sieglinde for her help and support and to grandma Maria, who created many of the beautiful handmade backgrounds. To Herbert who was always at hand to find the missing herbs when they were blossoming. Special thanks go to Helena, who was always helpful with scientific advice and difficult translations. To Don for his endless support, encouragement and stimulating advice. To Ulrich, Marianne, Klaus and Renate who showed us first-hand how vinegar is made from apple cider in large quantities and who happily answered all our detailed questions. We are eternally grateful to Tony for his support for our project — all the recipes were shot in his studio.

Our special thanks go to the wonderful team at Hardie Grant. To Fiona who introduced us, to Stephen and Kate who were very excited from the start about our vision for the book. To Kajal for her support, patience and timekeeping efforts and especially to Charlotte for the many edits and changes. Finally, thank you to Nicky for such a beautifully designed book. We are thrilled with how it looks — thank you so much.

ABOUT THE AUTHORS

Karin and Nici had to live apart in Austria (both in their vinegar socks and occasionally curd-lined) before they finally met in London, where they have worked together on an array of projects in Advertising, Photography and Illustration ever since.

Vinegar Socks by Karin Berndl and Nici Hofer

First published in 2015 by Hardie Grant Books

Hardie Grant Books (UK)
5th & 6th Floors
52-54 Southwark Street
London SE1 1UN
www.hardiegrant.co.uk

Hardie Grant Books (Australia)
Ground Floor, Building 1
658 Church Street
Melbourne, VIC 3121
www.hardiegrant.com.au

British Library Cataloguing-in-Publication Data. A catalogue
record for this book is available from the British Library.

ISBN: 978-1-78488-014-9

Publisher: Kate Pollard
Senior Editor: Kajal Mistry
Cover and Internal Design: Nicky Barneby
Photography: Karin Berndl and Nici Hofer
Copy Editor: Charlotte Coleman-Smith
Proofreader: Diana Vowles
Medical Advisor: Harriet Griffey
American Editor and Consultant: Denise Gibbon
Indexer: Cathy Heath
Colour Reproduction by p2d

Printed and bound in China by 1010

10 9 8 7 6 5 4 3 2 1